Stories in Mental Health:
Reflection, Inquiry, Action

Second Edition

Stories in Mental Health: Reflection, Inquiry, Action

Second Edition

Edited by Debra Nizette, Margaret McAllister and Peta Marks

ELSEVIER

ELSEVIER

Elsevier Australia. ACN 001 002 357
(a division of Reed International Books Australia Pty Ltd)
Tower 1, 475 Victoria Avenue, Chatswood, NSW 2067

ISBN: 978-0-7295-4395-8

> **Notice**
>
> Practitioners and researchers must always rely on their own experience and knowledge in evaluating and using any information, methods, compounds or experiments described herein. Because of rapid advances in the medical sciences, in particular, independent verification of diagnoses and drug dosages should be made. To the fullest extent of the law, no responsibility is assumed by Elsevier, authors, editors or contributors for any injury and/or damage to persons or property as a matter of products liability, negligence or otherwise, or from any use or operation of any methods, products, instructions, or ideas contained in the material herein.

National Library of Australia Cataloguing-in-Publication Data

A catalogue record for this
book is available from the
National Library of Australia

Senior Content Strategist: Libby Houston
Content Project Manager: Shubham Dixit
Edited by Caroline Hunter
Proofread by Tim Learner
Cover and internal design by Georgette Hall
Typeset by GW Tech Pvt. Ltd.
Printed in Singapore by Markono Print Media Pte Ltd

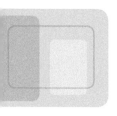

Contents

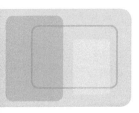

About the authors

Debra Nizette is a Credentialed Mental Health Nurse whose career has spanned clinical practice, education, leadership and consultancy. She has been an advisor in mental health nursing and an advocate for the consumer and their experience being the foundation for sound professional practice. Her role in policy development has promoted links to support consumer recovery through expert mental health nursing care.

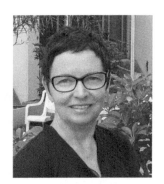

Margaret McAllister is Adjunct Professor of Nursing at Central Queensland University and a Credentialed Mental Health Nurse. She is an experienced researcher, with particular expertise in critical and narrative methods. Her collaborative research has spanned the impact of therapeutic interventions on wellbeing; an oral history of mental health nursing; and enhancing patient safety through evidence-based practice.

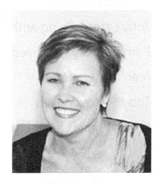

Peta Marks is a Credentialed Mental Health Nurse who works clinically in independent practice as a family and individual therapist for young people and their families. She has a successful consulting business working as a freelance mental health project manager, writer, editor and subject matter expert. Peta has a special interest and expertise in working with and writing about people who experience eating disorders and their families.

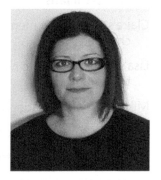

Acknowledgements

The authors would like to acknowledge the consumers, clinicians and carers who contributed their stories to the development of this resource. Your willingness to share your stories, your honesty and your openness have contributed to the potential of this resource to impact on the clinical practice of nurses and mental health nurses.

Todd Bagshaw

Bill Bailey

Rachael Bellair

Catherine Bennett

Colleen Blums

Lisa Bridle

Johanna Dalton

Amanda Davis

Zoe Farris

Carmel Flemming

Nadine Hedger

Jay Hendricks

Jarrad Hickmott

Anne Humbert

Claire Lees

Chris May

Jennifer McClay

Mike Musker

Louise O'Brien

Rachel Page

Elaine Painter

Christine Palmer

Jean Platts

Lyntara Quirke

Toby Raeburn

Jeremy Rodricks

Gordon Siebrecht

Kay Lillian Smith

Isabelle St Leon

Reg St Leon

Sonja St Leon

Makhala Swinson

Warren Ward

Bernie Waterhouse

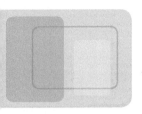

About this resource

This resource is structured into three parts. Part 1 provides an overview of the structure of the resource and outlines the processes of reflection, inquiry and action. Part 2 provides the foundational concepts for practice. Together, Parts 1 and 2 help the learner to engage with and make meaning of the stories for mental health nursing practice. The stories are presented in Part 3.

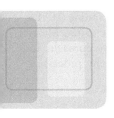

Part 1: Behind the scenes

OVERVIEW

This online resource contains video and audiofiles as well as transcripts of the stories and teaching activities and is divided into sections. Each video or audiofile is a story that conveys the mental health experiences of a consumer, carer or mental health nurse.

The aims of *Stories in Mental Health* are to bring learners close to people and their stories by hearing and observing, and to explore and understand their experiences, so that learners become informed and appreciative of the impact of mental health experiences on consumers, carers and clinicians.

This resource can be used online, by watching and listening to the videos and undertaking the activities online, or in hard copy format using the workbook and stories written as transcripts.

THE STORIES

This background information drives our approach to the resource. The stories—conveyed in videos, podcasts, photos, art and poems—speak for themselves. Rather than using actors and polished scripts, these stories are told by those who experienced them. We encourage you to fully experience and appreciate the stories they have to tell.

When an individual discusses their experience with mental disorder or the mental health system, we encourage you to understand that this is just one story. It does not necessarily define the person, or describe every mental health system. Most people whose stories are told here were not born with a mental disorder and their story of distress, or even recovery, is not, and will not be, their only life story. This is why we do not speak of a disorder as inherently part of who a person is. We do not call people 'schizophrenics' or 'anorexics', for example. Rather, we discuss the person first and their experiences with a mental health problem second. As such, we describe someone as a *person with* schizophrenia or a *person with* anorexia. Putting the person first is a practice that can benefit all mental health nurses. It

helps us to notice a person's humanity as well as their desires, drives and passions, well before we need to think about their strengths and deficits.

Another important point about 'story' is that strong narratives can drive people's lives almost continuously. People can, if reminded frequently enough, begin to see the disorder they are experiencing as inextricably tied to their identity. If this identity is non-productive, such as when a person who experienced child abuse continues to see themselves as a victim throughout adulthood, it can be a barrier to mental health and to the person flourishing in their life. In this resource you will meet people whose identity is no longer tied to a disorder label or who refuse the label attributed to them. We invite you to respect their position and to try to find meaning in the lessons they wish to impart.

One reason we have chosen these stories as learning and teaching tools is that powerfully told stories can convey lessons that are remembered for life. By encouraging our interviewees to put their experience into words, we have tried to transform the actual experience into a communicable representation of it. We have not recreated encounters; rather, we have asked people to reflect on their story and what was important about the story.

This process may help students of mental health to appreciate how people were affected by events emotionally, physically, psychologically and/or socially. It may also encourage students to reflect on the attitudes and skills that they still need to develop so that they can be therapeutic and helpful with consumers and carers they will meet in the future.

USING THE RESOURCE

Message to educators

We have designed a staged entry to the stories. After engaging with the emotion in the story, we invite learners to stand back from this affective aspect and try to reason through the complexities in the situation, so that they can imagine solutions and clarify how they intend to act in the future. We have thus included suggested activities for educators to encourage reflection, inquiry and action.

We encourage flexibility when using this resource in teaching and learning contexts. Sometimes you may wish to focus on one of the three components (reflection, inquiry, action) depending on the objective of your teaching and learning session, or you may wish to devise your own strategy based on the stories, identifying your own themes or learning needs.

Educators using this resource with nurses will need to have qualifications in mental health nursing. The theories developed by Peplau (theory of interpersonal relations), Altchul (nurse–patient relationship), Barker (the Tidal model), Travelbee (human-to-human relationship model) and other mental health nursing theorists help us to make meaning of the stories from the perspective of mental health nursing practice. This ensures that practice is embedded in the core values and concepts underpinning the profession. You may wish to undertake a separate session on nursing theorists before using this resource.

Reflection

Reflection is often assumed to be an inherent ability for students. However, we believe it is a learned cognitive skill and one that is key to professional practice. The power of reflection is harnessed throughout clinical supervision, because it assists in helping nurses to ensure that personal biases or ways of thinking are put to one side and a professional approach is used instead. In reflection, we often bring to the fore some of our values—and values guide action. By bringing values to the surface, they can be examined as to how they might facilitate or impede empathic relationships with others.

Students can be assisted to identify their values by noting how they feel while they are listening to a person recounting their story. Students can then self-scrutinise these values, by asking themselves whether their feelings would support or be a barrier to helping this individual or people like them.

We encourage you to remind learners that a value universal to mental health nurses is that we do not judge people. This is not our role. Rather, we aim to accept people and to convey to them unconditional, positive regard. If learners find that they are judging, they may benefit from being reminded to identify their personal biases and try to put them aside.

One way to deepen students' skills in reflection is to utilise Avis and Freshwater's (2006) three steps of reflection: reflection, attention and intention.

Another way to move from understanding at the individual level to the cultural level is to use Mezirow's (2000) transformative learning approach. In this view, reflection can focus on content, process or premise.

- In content reflection, we reflect on what we perceive or think about the situation. You could ask learners 'What was this story about?'
- In process reflection, we reflect on how situations unfold, or how interactions take place. You could ask learners 'How was this person feeling/acting?'
- In premise-based reflection, we develop an awareness of why the person, as part of a social or cultural group, perceives things or experiences things in the way that they do. This examination assists in questioning the social embeddedness and the equity or inequity of the experience. You could ask learners 'Is this experience a gendered or culture-based phenomenon?'

Finally, an easy-to-use communication framework that can assist students to listen to the stories and approach their analysis is Kanel's (2007) ABC framework. This involves:

A Attending to the person, by listening and being empathic.
B Breaking the problem down into manageable chunks, so that goal setting and change can be facilitated gradually.
C Exploring ways of coping. In difficult situations people cope in a variety of ways. It is important for students to understand the quality of the coping mechanism a person is displaying, because as a clinician they may decide to support the behaviour or gently reorient the person to take up some alternatives.

Note: In Part 2, Setting the scene, clinical supervision is discussed as essential to mental health nursing practice.

Inquiry

A pre-requisite for entering a story is listening. Listening is the basis of being able to truly hear someone's experience. It is from the story that our curiosity is ignited and our engagement with the person is made possible.

The next stage in inquiry is analysis—engaging in research and seeking out collateral information from a range of sources to help you become more informed about issues expressed in the story. In a one-on-one encounter you would prompt the person using a whole range of therapeutic communication techniques to go deeper into the story. From this informed perspective, key themes and issues emerge.

Action

The nurse's role in any therapeutic relationship is to be led by the consumer to facilitate safe and successful life transition. Nurses work in a variety of contexts, across the spectrum of prevention, treatment and support for wellbeing. This requires a range of therapeutic interventions and responses.

Nurses need to be able to work in a primary healthcare model and to transfer their health promotion and early-intervention techniques across lifespan, treatment and wellbeing spectrums. Nurses are not just illness-care workers, because mental health is not simply the absence of illness or disorder.

As the work in human flourishing allows us to see, wellbeing involves the holding of:

- positive emotions
- relationships
- meaning and purpose
- accomplishment.

Throughout the resource, we make suggestions as to how students can focus on developing these positive human attributes. For more information on this concept, go to Martin Seligman's homepage at Authentic Happiness.

Within this resource we invite learners to use reflection, inquiry and action to expand their therapeutic repertoire. This will assist them to be more flexible, creative, accountable and effective.

References

Avis M, Freshwater D 2006 Evidence for practice, epistemology, and critical reflection. Nursing Philosophy 7(4):216–224

Kanel K 2007 A guide to crisis intervention, 3rd edn. California State University, Fullerton

Mezirow J 2000 Learning as transformation. Jossey-Bass, San Francisco

Seligman M 2011 Flourish: a visionary new understanding of happiness and well-being. Free Press, New York.

Resources

Nursing Theories: **http://currentnursing.com/nursing_theory/interpersonal_theory.html**

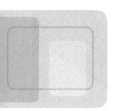

Part 2: Setting the scene
Getting ready to engage with the stories

We have identified a number of foundational concepts for practice that we believe need to be emphasised right at the very beginning. These are:

- resilience
- cultural and social inclusion
- being authentic
- the lived experience
- carers
- recovery
- clinical supervision.

Our hope is that after engaging in this resource, students will have greater appreciation for and skills to:

- be fully present with consumers and listen to their needs
- put aside their own concerns and personal dramas
- attend to each consumer's cultural uniqueness and be culturally safe
- understand what recovery means
- adopt an inclusive way of being with consumers, families and other clinicians
- continue to be therapeutic by accessing clinical supervision.

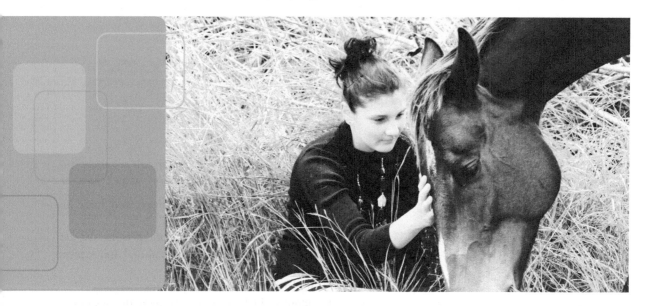

Makhala's story: Resilience

Introduction

Contemporary mental health nursing focuses on the person and their uniqueness. Although the person may, at some time, have been debilitated by an illness and have needed clinical care, they remain a human being with rights to autonomy and respect and with their own interests, abilities and contributions.

 View Makhala's story on evolve
http://evolve.elsevier.com/AU/Nizette/stories/

Reflection

Listen to Makhala's story, which was a healthcare experience that she recalls as good and bad.

1. How do you feel while listening to the story?
2. Makhala states that by helping other people she feels she is helping herself. Reflect on this statement. Reflect also on how listening to other people's stories can help you in your own life.

Inquiry

1. Makhala has integrated and transcended her adverse experience. Research the concept of resili-ence and identify characteristics of resilience that are relevant to Makhala.
2. One of the nurses took Makhala out to visit some horses, something the nurse knew was a passion for Makhala. What do you think was the impact of this action on Makhala's sense of self? In what way was it therapeutic?
3. How would you appraise the risks and benefits of this action?

Action

1. Explore the internet to locate a personal resilience or resilience assessment scale. How could you use this in practice?
2. Many people who work in nursing have experi-enced adversity. With consent, conduct an inter-view with a willing peer, using a resilience scale to determine the person's level of resilience.
3. What strategies could be implemented at various stages in the spectrum of interventions? (See Figure 1.)

The mental health nursing role is about working with people's strengths. In the primary healthcare context this may be about harnessing people's motivation to stay well. In the treatment context, this may be about reconnecting to strengths and shifting a focus from the deficits challenging their health to new strengths

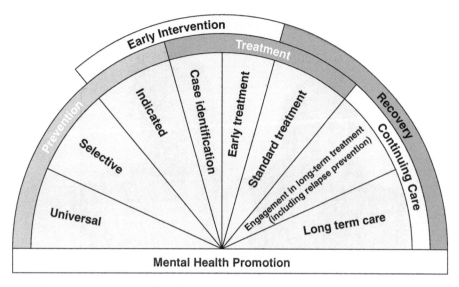

Figure 1 Spectrum of interventions for mental health
Source: www.health.gov.au/internet/main/publishing.nsf/content/A32F66862E8894ABCA25723E00175229/$File/prommon.
pdf.

that can be built upon to promote recovery and wellbeing.

Seligman's concept of PERMA helps synthesise and clarify aspects that promote wellbeing. Research **www.authentichappiness.sas.upenn.edu** to identify how those components are useful in practice.

Websites

Headspace: **www.headspace.org.au**
Inspire Foundation: **www.inspire.org.au**
Reachout: **www.reachout.com**
Young and Well Cooperative Research Centre:
    www.inspire.org.au/our-work/crc

Text links

Chapters 2, 9, 13 and 19 in Elder R, Evans K, Nizette D 2013 Psychiatric and mental health nursing, 3rd edn. Elsevier, Sydney.

References

Aronowitz T 2005 The role of 'envisioning the future' in the development of resilience among at-risk youth. Public Health Nursing 22:200–208

McAllister M, Lowe J 2011 The resilient nurse: empowering your practice. Springer, New York

A final word

Makhala has a joyful enthusiasm for life. But it hasn't always been this way. Although Makhala is young and her life, in many ways, is just starting out, she shows a strength of spirit and generosity by sharing her time, wisdom and compassion with other young people.

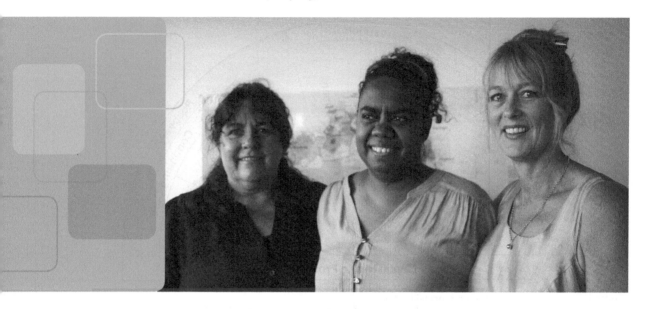

Jennifer, Anne and Christine: Cultural and social inclusion

Introduction

Anne Humbert was born in Katherine in the Northern Territory. She is a Mudburra woman on her mother's side and Ngarinman from her father's side. Christine May is a Wiradjuri woman born in Coonabarabran in New South Wales, and is descendant of John and Jessie May from the Aboriginal mission in Wellington and grandmother Katie May. Christine has worked for Queensland Health for almost 18 years. Both Anne and Christine work for the Cultural Healing Program on the Sunshine Coast as Indigenous Mental Health Workers.

Jennifer McClay was born on Yorta Yorta country, in the Wakool/Barham area in the Riverina. She is from Irish/English heritage and has worked as a mental health nurse for the past 33 years. She is an inaugural member of the Cultural Healing Program, which has been operating since 2002, and is the Clinical Nurse Consultant and Coordinator of the Program.

 View Jennifer, Anne and Christine's story on evolve http://evolve.elsevier.com/AU/Nizette/stories/

Videos

1. Working with Aboriginal people
2. Building trust and maintaining confidentiality
3. Listening to Aboriginal people's stories
4. The need for cultural healing

Reflection

1. Listen to the aspects about the work that the three clinicians find enjoyable and also notice the types of strategies they provide that are holistic.
2. What values do you feel are important for engaging with people's cultural identity?
3. How do these strategies add to the protective factors important to mental health and wellbeing for self and others?

Inquiry

1. Go to the Australian Indigenous Healthinfonet and click on the folder called 'Social and Emotional Wellbeing' to refresh your understanding of the holistic view of mental health that Indigenous people value as well as the factors occurring in everyday life that impact on Indigenous people's mental wellbeing. Why and how is culture important to understanding mental health in Indigenous people?

2. Take some time to explore this site and locate the assessment tools that have been tested to assure that they are culturally acceptable.

3. Trauma and loss are significant issues for Aboriginal people. Guidelines have been developed by expert clinicians that aim to be respectful of the cultural differences between Indigenous Australians and non-Indigenous Australians. Download the guidelines and use a highlighter pen to identify the specific issues that nurses should appreciate about unresolved emotional distress, its contribution to poor mental health and how nurses can behave to be respectful.

Action

If you work in nursing or a related field, find out where to locate the Aboriginal mental health workers who you can access in your practice. Share this information with your colleagues or make a laminated A4 poster to ensure that the information is communicated to everyone you work with.

Websites

AIHW: **www.aihw.gov.au/mental-health-indigenous**
Binan Goonj: **http://binangoonj.com.au**
Health Infonet: **www.healthinfonet.ecu.edu.au**
Indigenous Observatory: **www.aihw.gov.au/indigenous-observatory**

Text links

Chapters 6 and 7 in Elder R, Evans K, Nizette D 2013 Psychiatric and mental health nursing, 3rd edn. Elsevier, Sydney

References

Aboriginal Mental Health First Aid Training and Research Program 2008 Trauma and loss: guidelines for providing mental health first aid to an Aboriginal or Torres Strait Islander person. Orygen Youth Health Research Centre, University of Melbourne and beyondblue, Melbourne

Isaacs A, Pyett P, Oakley-Browne M, Gruis H, Waples-Crowe P 2010 Barriers and facilitators to the utilization of adult mental health services by Australia's Indigenous people: seeking a way forward. International Journal of Mental Health Nursing 19(2):75–82

Purdie N, Dudgeon P, Walker R (eds) 2010 Working together: Aboriginal and Torres Strait Islander mental health and wellbeing, principles and practice. Department of Health & Ageing, Canberra. Available at **www.ichr.uwa.edu.au/files/user5/Working_Together_book_web_0.pdf**

A final word

Christine states:

> Aboriginal people know when you're fair dinkum, it's just about listening, it's about respect, it's about being yourself really and people will know that. Don't be scared of Aboriginal people, there's nothing to be scared about, it's just about acknowledging them and the culture. Aboriginal people are loving people, kind people but we've also got an inbuilt fear and mistrust in us. Alleviate that and have fun with us and just enjoy being with an Aboriginal person … And wherever possible engage with an Aboriginal health worker whether it's a mental health worker or a generalist or a child worker, if you have to see an Aboriginal person and there's no Aboriginal health worker around just ask if there is an Aboriginal health worker in that district, would they please be able to come out with you and they'll probably really enjoy going out and will respect you more for asking them.

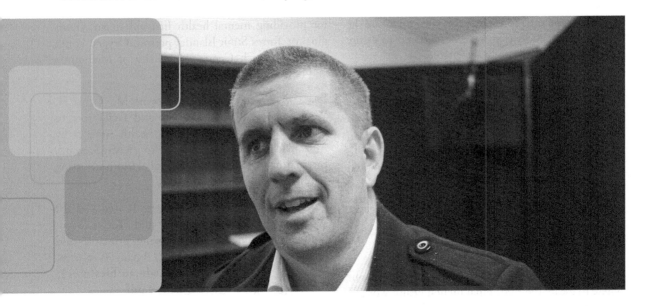

Toby's story: Being authentic

Introduction

Toby is a mental health nurse practitioner working in Sydney. He sees clients with complex mental health issues who are from vulnerable populations, often from CALD (culturally and linguistically diverse) backgrounds. Toby's way of working is to be engaging and real, to help the person to understand their own life and goals, and to hook them into services that can help provide stability, encouragement, support and direction.

View Toby's story on evolve
http://evolve.elsevier.com/AU/
Nizette/stories/

Reflection

1. Listen to Toby's experience and identify assumptions and actions unwittingly taken when we approach nursing from a monocultural perspective. Also listen to how Toby's way of working differs. What is it that Toby assumes, believes and practices that helps him to work effectively with vulnerable populations?

2. People from vulnerable groups may be more vulnerable to future traumas. Visiting a health professional should not be one of them. How can clinicians prevent re-traumatisation? How does past trauma manifest itself in people's lives?

Inquiry

According to the WHO Commission on Social Determinants of Health (2005), *social factors*—notably poverty, inequality, gender inequity, conflict and violence—are the major determinants of mental health and mental disorder. In Australia, there are several populations who experience more difficulties with these social factors.

1. Search the internet to find out which groups within Australia are most vulnerable. Mental Health in Multicultural Australia provides a good start.

2. To work effectively with vulnerable groups, nurses need to be culturally competent. Go to Chapter 6 in Elder, Evans and Nizette (2013) and read about strategies for culturally safe practice.

Action

1. Locate the Cultural Respect Framework developed by the South Australian government to promote Aboriginal and Torres Strait Islander

health. Make a poster or bookmark copy of the framework as an enduring gift for your classroom/clinical placement unit and for future learners.

2. Explain how trauma-informed care could be used in mental health nursing. Refer to **www.mhcc.org.au/TICP**.

Websites

Australian College of Mental Health Nurses: **www.acmhn.org**

Mental Health in Multicultural Australia: **www.mmha.org.au**

Mind Australia: **www.mindaustralia.org.au/index.htm**

Text links

Chapter 1, 2, 6, 7, 8 and 23 in Elder R, Evans K, Nizette D 2013 Psychiatric and mental health nursing, 3rd edn. Elsevier, Sydney

References

Australian Health Ministers' Advisory Council Standing Committee on Aboriginal and Torres Strait Islander Health Working Party (Comprising the Northern Territory, Queensland and South Australia) 2004 Cultural respect framework for Aboriginal and Torres Strait Islander health 2004–2009. AHMAC

Cross W, Bloomer M 2010 Extending boundaries: Clinical communication with culturally and linguistically diverse mental health clients and carers. International Journal of Mental Health Nursing 19(4):268–277

World Health Organization 2005–2008 Closing the gap in a generation: health equity through action on the social determinants of health. WHO, Geneva

A final word

Toby, as a nurse practitioner, is functioning at an advanced level and much of his expertise is now performed intuitively. But one important element of his way of working that we can all emulate is to practise authenticity, or 'being real', with clients. Toby doesn't pretend to be a person that he is not. He doesn't force his views or values onto others. Rather, he listens empathically and responds in a way that blends his unique personality with being concerned, hopeful and action-oriented towards the future.

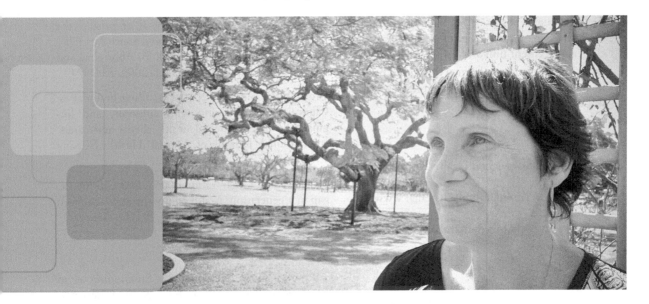

Bernie's story: The lived experience

Introduction

Bernie Waterhouse is a person with a lived experience of mental illness. At the peak of her career, when she held a managerial position in a large organisation, Bernie became psychotic. She was subsequently diagnosed with schizophrenia and hospitalised for almost six years.

View Bernie's story on evolve
http://evolve.elsevier.com/AU/Nizette/stories/

Reflection

1. How do you feel after listening to Bernie's story?
2. What do you think are her views about the meaning of recovery?
3. What is your perspective on recovery?

Inquiry

1. Why do you think a person who has a lived experience of schizophrenia (or any mental illness) could be a useful resource for mental health services?
2. Look at the National Mental Health Policy regarding consumer involvement consultants, personal helpers and mentors.

3. Look at the recovery star (see Figure 2), a resource that our UK colleagues routinely use, and consider how consumer involvement helps promote recovery.

Action

1. Listen to these podcasts on recovery and make a table comparing the recovery versus the medical model:
   a. Brenda Happell: **http://soundcloud.com/ipp-shr_podcasts_05/ippshr_podcast_050**
   b. SANE Australia, 'Getting better': **www.sane.org/information/factsheets-podcasts/207-getting-better**
2. How do you intend to demonstrate person-centred care in your interactions with consumers?

Websites

Recovery Innovations International Mental Health: **www.recoveryinnovations.com.au**
SANE Australia: **www.sane.org**

Text links

Chapters 2 and 15 in Elder R, Evans K, Nizette D 2013 Psychiatric and mental health nursing, 3rd edn. Elsevier, Sydney

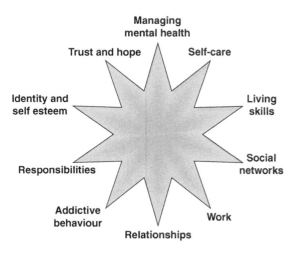

Figure 2 The recovery star
Source: www.imaginementalhealth.org.uk/_uploads/
Recovery%20STAR%20User%20Guide.pdf

References

Collier E 2010 Confusion of recovery: one solution. International Journal of Mental Health Nursing 19(1):16–21

Dornan DH, Felton C, Carpinello S 2000 Mental health recovery from the perspectives of consumer/survivors. Presentation at the American Public Health Association Annual Meeting, Boston. Available at **www.omh.ny.gov/omhweb/statewideplan/2006/html/chapter04.html**

A final word

Bernie's lived experience has given her unique insight into how nurses can make a constructive and positive impact through their work:

> Just always look for the little bit of light in that darkness and listen. Listen to what people are saying. Look at their verbal and nonverbal communication. Just believe in that person … believe that if they have the proper support and the proper care that they can move past the crisis. Remember that you are seeing them in crisis … you're not seeing the person as they really are.

> Mental illness is only a part of that person and often only for a limited amount of time, when they are having that episode. So look for the light and believe in their ability to move towards wellness.

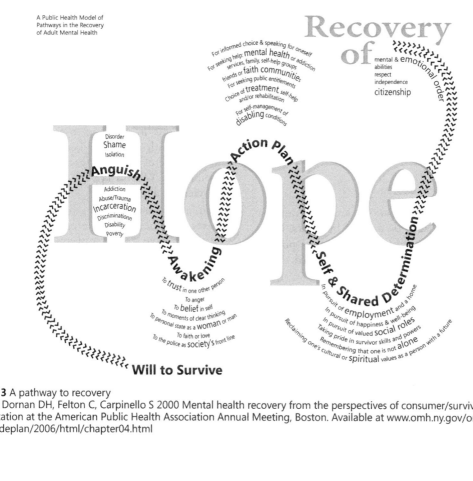

Figure 3 A pathway to recovery
Source: Dornan DH, Felton C, Carpinello S 2000 Mental health recovery from the perspectives of consumer/survivors. Presentation at the American Public Health Association Annual Meeting, Boston. Available at www.omh.ny.gov/omhweb/statewideplan/2006/html/chapter04.html

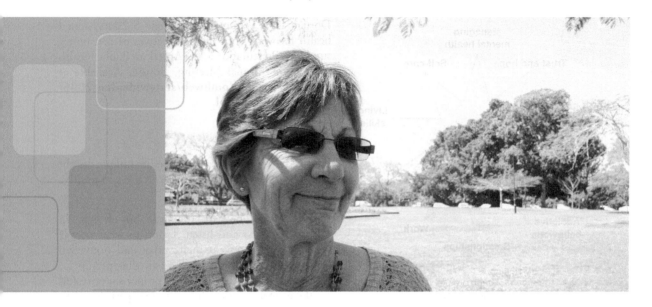

Jean's story: Carers

Introduction

As well as being the primary carer of her adult son, Daniel, who has schizophrenia, Jean Platts has been involved in the carer's arm of ARAFMI Queensland since 1999 and is the Queensland carer representative on the National Mental Health Consumer & Carer Forum. Jean is passionate about issues associated with rehabilitation and enabling people with mental illness to live productive, satisfying and independent lives.

Quick facts

There are several organisations around Australia that are either managed by or used by carers. Only recently has the important role that carers play in supporting consumers been acknowledged. One definition of a carer is:

> A person of any age who, without being paid, cares for another person who needs ongoing support because of a long-term medical condition, a mental illness, a disability, frailty or the need for palliative care. A carer may or may not be a family member and may or may not live with the person. Volunteers under the auspices of a voluntary organisation are not included (Queensland Health 2007).

View Jean's story on evolve
http://evolve.elsevier.com/AU/Nizette/stories/

Reflection

1. Jean talks about becoming a consumer herself at one time, in response to the many stressors involved with caring for her son. In what way did the role of a carer impact on Jean and those around her? What is a carer's role in recovery? Is it different to a nurse's role?

2. Jean invites nurses to do more than just 'tick boxes and checklists'. She encourages nurses to sit down, have a chat, converse with consumers. Reflect on some of the ways you could ensure that you do this in your clinical practice. Identify some of the potential barriers to this type of activity and how you might resolve them.

Inquiry

1. Jean talks about the concept of 'inclusion'. What does this term mean? How is that enacted during the assessment of a client, and then in collaborative goal-setting and in shared decision making?

2. How do you balance the right of the person to make their own decisions with the need to include families and carers in that collaborative relationship?

3. Explore the literature on psychosocial disability. How are carers identified in the literature?

Action

1. Stigma is a key issue for people who experience mental health issues and their carers. Jean talks about systemic, individual and consumer/carer-centred stigma. Differentiate between these types of stigma.

2. An assignment topic on this issue could be: Research the literature on the primary healthcare approach and psychosocial disability. Discuss how a primary healthcare approach can impact on psychosocial disability.

3. Jean asks that nurses be inclusive of carers in their practice. From your observations of practice and research, identify behaviours and practices that include carers. Locate and read the policy statements (practice or service) in your health service area that support carer inclusion.

Websites

ARAFMI Australia: **www.arafmiaustralia.asn.au**
Fountain House: **www.fountainhouse.org**
International Journal of Mental Health Nursing: **http://au.wiley.com/WileyCDA/WileyTitle/productCd-INM.html**

Journal of Psychosocial Nursing: **www.healio.com/journals/jpn**
National Mental Health Consumer & Carer Forum: **www.nmhccf.org.au**
Stepping Stone Clubhouse: **www.steppingstoneclubhouse.org.au**
The Richmond Fellowship: **www.rfnsw.org.au**

Text links

Chapters 9 and 25 in Elder R, Evans K, Nizette D 2013 Psychiatric and mental health nursing, 3rd edn. Elsevier, Sydney

References

National Mental Health Consumer & Carer Forum 2012 What mental health consumers and carers want. Available at **www.nmhccf.org.au/documents/What%20C%20&%20C%20want%20brochure%20-%20web%20version.pdf**

Queensland Health 2007 Queensland Government Carer Recognition Policy. Queensland Health, Brisbane

A final word

Jean's voice as a carer and a mother needs to be heard. We are so grateful to her for sharing the aspirations she has for her son, and to learn from her that when a child develops a serious mental illness, families can adapt and can be resilient.

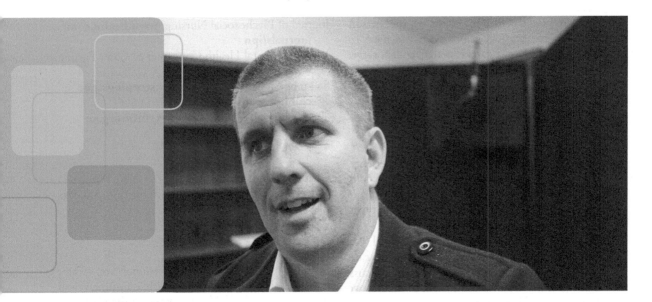

Recovery

Introduction

There are several references to the concept of recovery in the resource. You have met Toby previously. In this excerpt, Toby talks about his perspective on recovery and how it has helped to reorient his practice over the past 10–15 years.

 View Toby's story on evolve
http://evolve.elsevier.com/AU/
Nizette/stories/

Reflection

Listen to Toby's story. He says that 20 years ago 'patients' wouldn't have been 'allowed' to go off their medication, to stop seeing their psychiatrist or to attend university. How has the system changed to support the recovery focus?

Inquiry

How has the scope of practice of mental health nurses changed over the past 20 years?

Action

Locate a mental health nursing article written in the 1980s and compare the nurse's role then to the current literature on recovery.

Websites

National Coalition for Mental Health Recovery: **http://ncmhr.org**
The Tidal model: **www.tidal-model.com**

Text links

Chapters 2, 3, 4, 5 and 6 in Elder R, Evans K, Nizette D 2013 Psychiatric and mental health nursing, 3rd edn. Elsevier, Sydney

References

Mental Health Coordinating Council. Mental health recovery philosophy into practice: a workforce development guide. Available at **www.mhcc.org.au/ resources/staff-development-guide.aspx**

Rickwood D 2006 Pathways of recovery: 4As framework for preventing further episodes of mental illness. Commonwealth of Australia, Canberra

A final word

Toby states:

> It's an exciting time to be part of mental health nursing, the sky's the limit. I mean innovation is happening all around us and it's going to be fun to meet you.

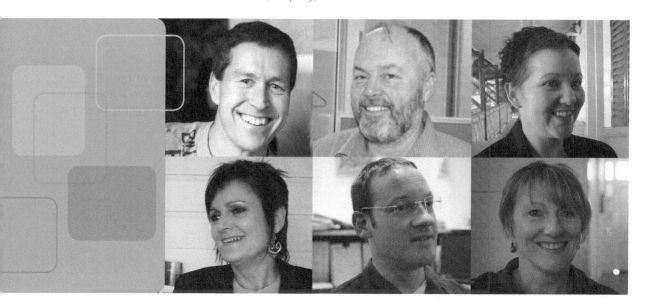

Clinical supervision: Learning about self and others

Introduction

All of the clinicians interviewed for this resource identified the central role that clinical supervision has for them, the benefits they experience from undertaking it and the elements that they believe are most important. Listen to the collective voices of the mental health nurses as they discuss what clinical supervision means to them.

View this story on evolve
http://evolve.elsevier.com/AU/
Nizette/stories/

What you need to know

In Australia, 'clinical supervision' is the term used to support the professional practice development of mental health nurses. It is a structured arrangement whereby two or more nurses formally meet to reflect and review clinical situations. It provides time out from constant practice and an opportunity to engage in guided and critical reflection on practice with an experienced practitioner. The aim is to support the clinician in their professional environment in order to enhance care for consumers and professional capability.

Major assumptions underpinning the effectiveness of supervision are that:

- self-awareness is enhanced, and this is key to being able to help others
- by discussing puzzles, problems and ethical dilemmas, new approaches or strategies may be developed
- sharing concerns provides an opportunity to vent stress, be specific about examples of consumer resistances or alleviate worrying obstacles such as transference.

Reflection

Psychoanalytic theory is one of the earliest theories to understand the human mind, and a very important component of this therapeutic approach was for clinicians to have undergone their own therapy. This assists in developing self-knowledge. With self-awareness, the assumption was that the clinician could better engage in an empathic and helpful relationship with others.

Proctor (1986) provides a widely adopted model of supervision that comprises three elements:

a. *normative:* adherence to standards of the profession

b. *formative:* provides opportunity for skills and knowledge development

c. *restorative:* assists in the understanding and managing of emotional stress in nursing.

1. Think about a situation where you weren't able to fully engage or empathise with a client. What were the barriers limiting your therapeutic effectiveness? Organise them into Proctor's three elements.

2. Refer to the article by Brunero and Stein-Parbury (2008) to identify positive outcomes of clinical supervision using Proctor's model.

3. Consider which of the reported outcomes in Table 1 in the article may have been useful to you in a clinical supervision session.

4. How could the positive outcomes of Proctor's model have helped you to identify new strategies or approaches?

Inquiry

Clinical supervision has a long history in mental health. Explore the origins of how self-exploration was utilised across time, and how this is relevant to current clinical practice.

Action

1. Provide a one-sentence definition for the following terms:

    transference
    countertransference
    restorative
    normative
    reflection
    debriefing
    unconscious
    devil's advocate
    peer supervision
    group supervision
    one-to-one supervision
    supervision process toolbox
    Berg's (1984) EARS solution-focused technique
    catharsis

2. Watch the episode of 'In treatment' at **www.youtube.com/watch?v=KajVjF25qRg** where Paul, the therapist, accesses clinical supervision from Gina. How does Gina focus her questions to prompt reflection in Paul?

3. What new insights do you think Paul begins to appreciate having had this conversation with Gina?

4. What value do you think supervision served for Paul?

5. What are the risks of clinical supervision?

6. How is the therapist assisted to reflect on his own unconscious or unarticulated reactions?

Website

Australian College of Mental Health Nurses: **www.acmhn.org/career-resources/clinical-supervision.html**

Text links

Chapters 1, 5, 17, 19 and 22 in Elder R, Evans K, Nizette D 2013 Psychiatric and mental health nursing, 3rd edn. Elsevier, Sydney

References

Australian College of Mental Health Nurses 2002 Clinical supervision models, measures and practice. ACMHN, Canberra. Available at **www.acmhn.org/images/stories/Media/Monographs/pub_monograph_2002.pdf**

Australian College of Mental Health Nurses 2010 Standards of practice for Australian mental health nurses, 2010. ACMHN, Canberra

Berg I 1994 Family-based services: a solution focused approach. Norton, New York

Brunero S, Stein-Parbury J 2008 The effectiveness of clinical supervision in nursing: an evidenced based literature review. Australian Journal of Nursing 25(3):86–94

Proctor B 1986 Supervision: a cooperative exercise in accountability. In: Marken M, Payne M (eds) Enabling and ensuring. Leicester National Youth Bureau and Council for Education and Training in Youth and Community Work, Leicester, pp 21–23

A final word

Christine states:

> I think that anyone working in the field of mental health needs to have clinical supervision. I think it's important for novices *and* experts, because it's about reflecting on your practice and being thoughtful about working with people, and it keeps you much more honest and professional.

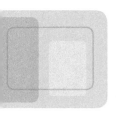

Part 3: Stories from consumers, carers and clinicians

This resource has made a concerted attempt to use stories from people's real-life experiences, including consumers, carers and clinicians. Stories have a power that is unique. Through listening to someone's story you can appreciate what it feels like in a subjective and close way, rather than what it looks like in an objective and dispassionate way.

Stories can move people towards action, rather than simple understanding. Since nursing is a practice, we aim to assist learners to put lessons into practice, not just to know facts. For stories to reveal their powerful messages you need to be ready to participate fully in the storytelling process. This is why we ask you to reflect, inquire and act in relation to each of the stories.

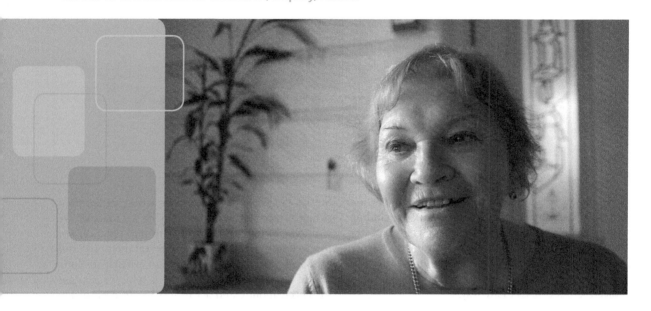

Claire's story: How mental health has changed

Introduction

Claire Lees is a retired mental health nurse and very proud of it. She trained between 1960 and 1963 at Claybury Hospital, a large psychiatric hospital in England—something Australian psychiatric hospitals were modelled after. Claire describes the hospital like a city on its own. It covered about 50 square kilometres and on the land was a farm, a butchery, cricket pitches, football fields, a large kitchen, a medical unit and a dentist. Claire remembers only one rule: when you left the premises you had to leave the large key that unlocked every door and was fitted around your waist at the sentry box.

View Claire's story on evolve
http://evolve.elsevier.com/AU/
Nizette/stories/

Videos

1. A day in the life
2. The paradigm shift
3. What I value about mental health nursing

Reflection

1. Engage in an interview analysis, using three steps of reflection: reflection, attention and intention (Avis & Freshwater, 2006).
   a. What are the main issues raised about changes in mental health nursing?
   b. Imagine you are being interviewed on the future of mental health nursing. What main issues will you raise?
2. Cicero, the great Roman orator, once said: 'Those who do not know their past will forever remain children.' Relating this quote to nursing, what lessons from the past in mental health nursing do you think need to be heard to assist nurses to 'grow up' professionally?

Inquiry

1. Claybury Hospital was one of many asylums built in the 19th century. Perform an internet search to understand the history of this institution at: **www. reptonparkwoodfordgreen.co.uk/rp_history.htm**.
2. What does 'asylum' mean and how would this have been achieved in the hospital where Claire worked?
3. There are many examples of asylums in Australia. Find some images or virtual museums of institutions in your state.

4. The history of psychiatric care dates a long way back. To trace this history, view the short presentation at this site: **www.rcpsych.ac.uk/training/students/historyofpsychiatry.aspx**.

5. Claire describes the rituals of daily working life for nurses and patients living in an asylum. Make a list of what was mentioned and what you think would need to be done in the running of a major precinct housing 2000 patients and hundreds of staff.

6. You will notice that Claire uses the term 'patient'; what other terms are you aware of that might be used, and why?

7. In the early days of psychiatry, efforts to calm and contain patients were many. Compare and contrast strategies used 50–100 years ago with those used today. Try to find good and bad examples.

8. Around the time when Claire was training, a major paradigm shift was occurring in the treatment of mental disorders in the developed world. What was this, and what did it lead to?

9. How do you think the paradigm shift impacted on the role of nurses? How did they spend their time before this innovation, and how did they spend their time afterwards?

10. One key difference about nursing practice then and now is that today promotion of wellbeing helps to prevent the development of mental disorders; and early intervention, through assertive treatments and monitoring, promotes active recovery. What prevention and recovery practices were overlooked in those early days of psychiatry?

Action

1. Journal how the knowledge and insights from this chapter might impact on your current clinical practice.

2. Suggested assignment topic: According to Helman (1990), rituals serve a very important function for human society. They can be grounding, offering a sense of purpose and social connection, keeping a person in touch with core values, humanity, god and life. Arguably, ritual activities are no longer highly valued in modern society. Catanzaro (2002) contends that with the rise of technical rationalism, ritual has been dismissed as belonging to the primitive. In contemporary health practice, ritual mostly has a negative connotation—it is associated with irrationality and thoughtless repetition, perpetuating habit rather than reason, and propping up traditions that prevent advancement. But living daily life without ritual and tradition can also reduce meaning and succour. What are your thoughts on this debate? How will it shape your future practice?

Website

Movement for Global Mental Health: **www.globalmentalhealth.org**

Text links

Chapters 2, 3, 5 and 8 in Elder R, Evans K, Nizette D 2013 Psychiatric and mental health nursing, 3rd edn. Elsevier, Sydney

References

Avis M, Freshwater D 2006 Evidence for practice, epistemology, and critical reflection. Nursing Philosophy 7(4):216–224

Catanzaro AM 2002 Beyond the misapprehension of nursing rituals. Nursing Forum 37:17–27

Helman C 1990 Culture, health and illness. Butterworth-Heinemann, Oxford

Ion M, Beer D 2003 Valuing the past: the importance of an understanding of the history of psychiatry for healthcare professionals, service users and carers. International Journal of Mental Health Nursing 12(4):237–242

Madsen W, McAllister M, Godden J, Greenhill J, Reed R 2009 Nursing's orphans: how the system of nursing education in Australia is undermining professional identity. Contemporary Nurse 32(1):9–18

A final word

Claire provides some motivating words for students:

I think if anybody wants to become a mental health nurse, go for it. It's the best profession because you're always thinking, you're always learning … no two people are the same, you've got their diagnosis but you've also got the person's personality, and it's always a challenge.

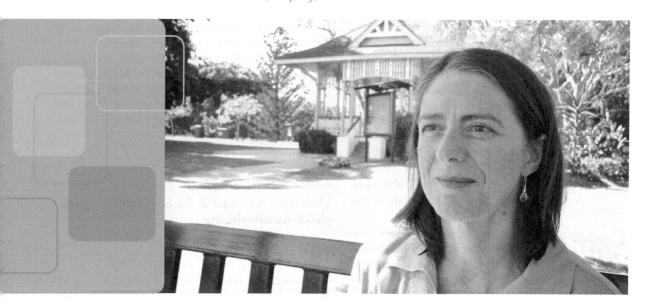

Lisa's story: Experiencing a major life transition

Introduction

Lisa is a social worker and mother of three children: Amelia, Sean and Declan. Sean has Down syndrome. He's 16 years old and in Year 10 at a private Catholic boys' school. He dreams about jobs, girlfriends and moving out of home. He's got a great sense of humour and an ordinary adolescent attitude. He experiences rejection at times and isn't able to communicate very well about his feelings or experiences. But he's got a fantastic enthusiasm about him; he loves camping, he goes tandem bike riding with his dad and, when he's interested in something, he just absolutely embraces it with a great passion.

What you need to know

Lisa's story raises awareness about two major issues:

- the experience of raising a child with a disability
- the importance of perinatal and infant mental health.

About 5% of Australian children have some type of disability (AIHW, 2004). Their parents are dealing with a range of emotions, but most adapt with help and support from the community. Lisa recounts that the events surrounding Sean's birth were traumatising for her and her family.

Listening to the story, you will hear Lisa describe shock, guilt, isolation and fear. Unfortunately, there were times when Lisa experienced unhelpful encounters with clinicians. While this is disappointing, we can learn from Lisa's story about what mothers, families and infants need during such a critical time.

Had Lisa been able to access best practice in infant mental health, she may well have had her traumatic experience alleviated and been given timely support to make a successful transition to being a mother and carer for a child born with a disability. As it happens, Lisa has successfully negotiated the challenges and is now the mother of a happy and healthy family.

 View Lisa's story on evolve
http://evolve.elsevier.com/AU/
Nizette/stories/

Videos

1. My son's birth—a difficult time for me and others
2. A story of personal and family coping

Reflection

Reflect on the following comment Lisa made in the extended version of this interview. How will you protect yourself against losing 'kindness'?

So what would have helped, from a health professional point of view, is that I needed people to be really positive and I needed people to be really kind. I was aware that people aren't always just comfortable with disability and that's okay, but I think sometimes it would have helped if people had educated themselves about the potential in the lives of people with disability, rather than going on outdated stereotypes of what is possible—and as one of my friends said, 'Just don't be bastards, don't be mean, don't be kind of running around trying to impress us with your knowledge or your power, just be kind.'

Inquiry

The World Association for Infant Mental Health explains that mental healthcare before, during and after pregnancy is vital for the infant–family system. Mental health nurses appreciate that a child's social-emotional development is as important as their brain and physical development, and it is vital to support the family's mental health and wellbeing during the challenging life transition of child birth.

Babies and young children thrive when they are cared for by adults who are deeply engaged with them. Responsive relationships with consistent primary caregivers help build positive attachments that support healthy social-emotional development. Adults in this context will also thrive if their resilience stores are renewed and the major life transition of child-raising is supported.

1. Listen to Lisa's experiences and identify the resilience stores that operated or could have operated throughout the intensive care experience. Research and share a clear definition of infant mental health and what its objectives are.
2. Lisa's feelings of guilt and depression were at times overwhelming. Try to practise the ABC framework for therapeutic engagement. If you were in the video, listening to Lisa, how would you aim to Attend, Break the problem down and facilitate Coping?

Action

1. Listen to Lisa's story, making notes as you go, using a framework of appreciative inquiry (AI) as outlined in the Resources section (see below).
2. Research the three different subtypes of Down syndrome. Chapter 12 in Elder, Evans and Nizette (2013) provides some information and

there are state-based associations to be found on the Web (see below).
3. Research and locate the local service for perinatal and infant mental health that exists in your district. Store the contact details for your professional practice.

Websites

Down Syndrome Association of Western Australia: **http://dsawa.asn.au**
Down Syndrome Association Queensland: **www.dsaq.org.au**
Down Syndrome NSW: **www.dsansw.org.au/index.php**
Down Syndrome Victoria: **www.downsyndromevictoria.org.au**
National Centre for Infants, Toddlers and Families: **www.zerotothree.org**
Queensland Parents for People with a Disability: **www.qppd.org**
Raising Children Network: **http://raisingchildren.net.au/articles/raising_a_child_with_a_disability.html**
World Association for Infant Mental Health: **www.waimh.org/i4a/pages/index.cfm?pageid=1**

Table 1 Assumptions underpinning appreciative inquiry

AI is based on assumptions that:
In every society, organisation or group, something works
What we focus on becomes our reality
Reality is created in the moment, and there are multiple realities
The art of asking questions of an organisation or a group influences the group in some way
People have more confidence and comfort to journey to the future (the unknown) when they carry forward parts of the past (the known)
If we carry parts of the past forward, they should be what is best about the past
It is important to value differences
The language we use creates our reality

Source: Carter B 2007 Working it out together: being solution-focused in the way we nurse with children and their families. In: McAllister M (ed.) Solution-focused nursing. Palgrave, Basingstoke, pp 63–76.

Resources

Appreciative inquiry is a framework for thinking appreciatively with people about situations and settings. It is well-established as a way of bringing about organisational change and is becoming established as a way of guiding research. It also has many positive elements to offer nurses working with children and their families. These connections are explored, drawn out and contrasted with the more dominant problem-oriented discourses.

AIHW 2004 Children with disabilities in Australia. Cat. no. DIS 38. AIHW, Canberra

Carter B 2005 'They've got to be as good as mum and dad': children with complex health care needs and their siblings' perceptions of a Diana Community Nursing Service. Clinical Effectiveness in Nursing 9(2):49–61

Carter B 2006 'One expertise among many'; working appreciatively to make miracles instead of finding problems: using appreciative inquiry as a way of reframing research. Journal of Research in Nursing 11(1):48–63

Cooperrider DL, Whitney D 1999 Appreciative inquiry: a positive revolution in change. In Holman P, Devane T (eds) The change handbook: group methods for shaping the future. Berrett-Koehler Publishers, San Francisco, CA

Hammond S 1998 The thin book of appreciative inquiry, 2nd edn. Thin Book Publishing, Plano, TX

Text links

Chapters 9, 12 and 25 in Elder R, Evans K, Nizette D 2013 Psychiatric and mental health nursing, 3rd edn. Elsevier, Sydney

References

AIHW 2004 Children with disabilities in Australia. Cat. no. DIS 38. AIHW, Canberra

Carter B 2007 Working it out together: being solution-focused in the way we nurse with children and their families. In: McAllister M (ed.) Solution-focused nursing. Palgrave, Basingstoke, pp 63–76

Pannen I 2011 'What will I do?' Depression and the trick to keep breathing. Mental Health Review Journal 16(3):113–117

A final word

Lisa states:

> One of the things I remember about the early months of Sean's life is just the number of medical appointments that we had and the sheer number of people who we had to interact with and the hours that we spent waiting at hospital outpatients appointments where the rooms were never set up, there were never ever change tables, there was always a lack of space … I had my daughter there as well, trying to entertain her for hours on end. We would literally spend hours waiting and then kind of five minutes with the doctor, generally getting bad news …

> I think it's just important for health professionals to know that that is your experience and how exhausting it is. You don't need people being very officious, you just need people to be really kind of understanding and flexible and to do what they can to make it, at least, a less horrendous experience.

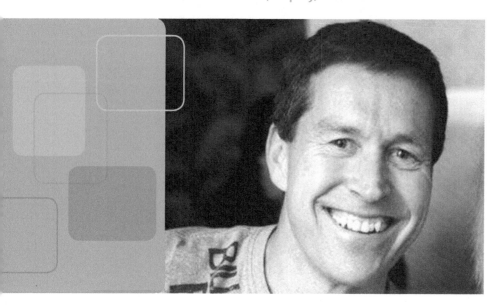

Mike's story: Facilitating empowerment

Introduction

Mike Musker is a clinical nurse consultant at the Forensic Mental Health Service of South Australia and Associate Lecturer at Flinders University and the University of Adelaide. For many years he has worked with people who have an intellectual disability.

 View Mike's story on evolve
http://evolve.elsevier.com/AU/
Nizette/stories/

Reflection

1. Listen to the podcast and reflect on what Mike finds rewarding about his work. Discuss this with a peer and develop a critical position on this issue.
2. Learning disability is a social construct: what does this mean?
3. How has the meaning of this changed practice over time?

Inquiry

Nurses working in the specialised area of intellectual disability are particularly focused on supporting clients to live happy, connected, fulfilling lives.

Maslow's hierarchy of needs provides a useful framework to understand what people's needs are and how nurses can work to meet these needs. Use Figure 4 to map the practices and concerns that Mike and his colleagues use to support the person and their family to achieve a high quality of life.

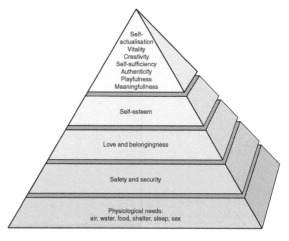

Figure 4 Maslow's hierarchy of needs
Source: http://intuitiontellsmeso.wordpress.com/2009/08/19/
problemnegative-thought-patterns-becoming-aware/
maslows-hierarchy/

Action

- **DRAG and DROP 1**

  Fit the behaviours with the unmet need:

  harm to others
  threatening
  hostile
  self-harming
  bite themselves
  washing and dressing
  poor patterns of sleep
  mood disruption
  lack of control over eating
  medications that impede eating
  gagging
  constipation
  overactivity
  underactivity
  social skills deficit
  sexuality

- **DRAG and DROP 2**

  Fit the behaviours that clinicians and carers might use that impede the person's ability to meet their needs:

  talking down to the person
  ignoring physical cues
  failing to protect the person from humiliation
  limiting and controlling behaviours that you have
      no right to control
  failing to acknowledge the need for companion-
      ship
  overlooking the need for someone to be involved
      in productive activity
  imposing a routine on to the person regardless of
      their preferences and patterns
  not balancing respect for independence with the
      need to facilitate social acceptability

Websites

AIHW: **www.aihw.gov.au/publication-detail/?id=6442468183**
Clinicians Knowledge Network: **http://health.qld.campusguides.com/perinatal-infant-mentalhealth**

Mental Health Professionals Network: **www.mhpn.org.au/News/Events/tabid/201/agentType/View/PropertyID/29/Default.aspx**
Women's and Children's Health Network: **www.cyh.com/HealthTopics/HealthTopicDetails.aspx?p=114&np=306&id=1876**

Text links

Chapters 12, 22 and 23 in Elder R, Evans K, Nizette D 2013 Psychiatric and mental health nursing, 3rd edn. Elsevier, Sydney

References

Bell R 2012 'Does he have sugar in his tea?' Communication between people with learning disabilities, their carers and hospital staff. Tizard Learning Disability Review 17(2):57–63

Musker M 2007 Learning disabilities and solution focused nursing. In McAllister M (ed) Solution focused nursing: rethinking practice. Macmillan-Palgrave, London

Harvey ST, Fisher LJ, Green VM 2012 Evaluating the clinical efficacy of a primary care-focused, nurse-led, consultation liaison model for perinatal mental health. International Journal of Mental Health Nursing 21(1):75–81

Taua C, Hepworth J, Neville C 2012 Nurses' role in caring for people with a comorbidity of mental illness and intellectual disability: a literature review. International Journal of Mental Health Nursing 21(2):163–174

A final word

Mike makes working in the highly specialised environment of forensic mental health nursing look easy. The way he works with clients who have special needs because of profound intellectual disability is transferable to every context where nurses work: this is about understanding a person's likes and dislikes, and supporting them to live in ways that are rewarding socially, psychologically and spiritually. Working mindfully with people is challenging, rewarding and inspiring.

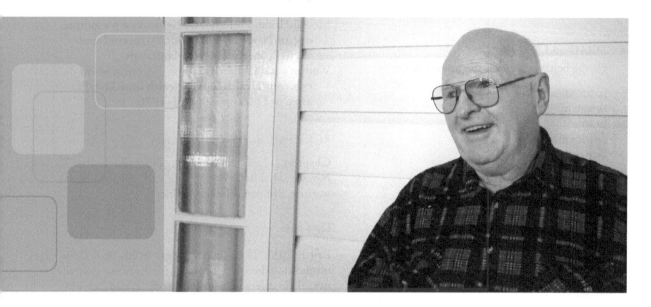

Gordon's story: Fatherhood

Introduction

Gordon is the proud father of Pamela and two other children. Gordon is a retired construction manager and the coordinator of Minders, a Brisbane-based support group for fathers of children with mental health issues. He has strong beliefs about what parenting means, and particularly the role of fathers.

Several years ago, as an adolescent, Pamela experienced several episodes of schizophrenia but is now well into her journey of recovery. Gordon reflects on Pamela's strength and resilience and shares insights about ways that health professionals can better relate and connect with families—who are, or can be, productive partners in care.

 View Gordon's story on evolve
http://evolve.elsevier.com/AU/
Nizette/stories/

Videos

1. Relating with carers
2. Family coping and caring

3. Gobbledygook
4. A father's reflection

Reflection

1. Notice how some consumers and carers, rather than seeking out information for themselves, rely on the information provided to them by health professionals.
2. Society has tended to view that mothers have the most influence on their children's mental health, growth and development, but Gordon reminds us of the importance of considering the role and needs of fathers. What messages do you hear from Gordon's comments?
3. Make a list of the range of beliefs and emotions felt and expressed in this family.

Inquiry

1. Investigate the websites provided (see below) to consider how they might act as an empowering resource for families. Also consider their limitations.

2. What is it that the interpersonal communication and support from a health professional can offer that a website may not?

Action

1. Locate for your service the most recent policy documents to enhance carer participation in health service delivery.
2. Consider what Gordon says about the importance of clear, jargon-free language. Next time you are in a situation where you are able to listen to a health professional relating to a family member, make a note of how many jargon words are used in the interaction. Then make a note of how these terms could be replaced with plain English.

Websites

ARAFMI Qld: **www.arafmiqld.org**
blueVoices: **www.beyondblue.org.au/index. aspx?link_id=3**
Carers Australia: **http://carersaustralia.com.au**
Consumers Health Forum of Australia: **www.chf. org.au**
GROW Australia: **www.grow.net.au**
Mental Health Carers Arafmi Australia: **www. arafmiaustralia.asn.au**
Mental Health Council of Australia: **www.mhca. org.au**
National Mental Health Consumer & Carer Forum: **www.nmhccf.org.au**

Private Mental Health Consumer Carer Network (Australia): **http://pmha.com.au/pmhccn/ Home.aspx**

Text links

Chapters 24 and 25 in Elder R, Evans K, Nizette D 2013 Psychiatric and mental health nursing, 3rd edn. Elsevier, Sydney

Reference

Kertchok R, Yunibhand J, Chaiyawat W 2011 Creating a new whole: helping families of people with schizophrenia. International Journal of Mental Health Nursing 20(1):38–46

A final word

Gordon says:

> The key messages would be to listen to the carers, respond in simple English not medical terms, make certain that the person that you're talking to has picked up the message you're trying to explain, what the medical staff are going to be doing with the person that you're caring for, to listen to both parties of a family, which is the mother and the father, and also consider what effect this will have on the siblings of the person, because sometimes those siblings may be helpful in assisting the person that's suffering.

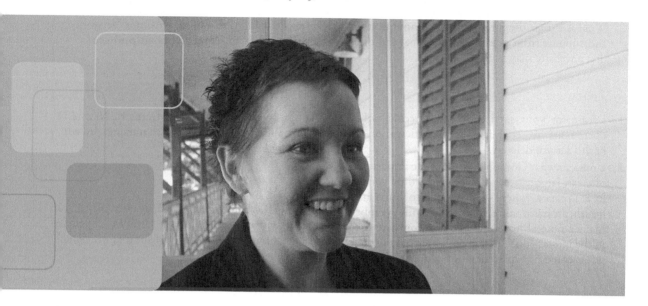

Rachel's story: Relating to young people

Introduction

Rachel is a mental health nurse who specialises in child and youth work. Providing mental healthcare to children and young people is vital. Current thinking in mental health is that early intervention in young people could actually prevent the onset of full-blown disorders and enhance the person's resilience to stressors that would otherwise make them vulnerable to illness. As Rachel explains, there are some issues and skills required that are specific to this population. Working with young people is also particularly rewarding.

View Rachel's story on evolve
http://evolve.elsevier.com/AU/
Nizette/stories/

Videos

1. Assessment issues in child and youth mental health
2. Young people and identity
3. Consent and confidentiality

Reflection

Consider this inspirational quote: 'We must view young people not as empty bottles to be filled but as candles to be lit.' How may good clinicians orientate their practice to fulfil this aim?

Inquiry

1. What do you understand to be some of the protective factors that can be noticed and developed by nurses working with children and young people?
2. What risk factors are associated with childhood and adolescence?
3. Adolescence involves a life transition, where one begins to break away from an earlier life phase that is typically characterised as one of dependence on adults and compliance with directions; and a trialling of a new independence in thinking and behaviour. How does Rachel say she balances the challenge of respecting a young person's growing independence, while acknowledging the rights of parents and care givers?
4. Find out about the Gillick competence. Why would nurses working with young people need to have a good understanding of what this is and how to use it?

Action

1. Adolescence is a turbulent time for young people. It involves a lot of change, and transition can

require that you move from one set of coping mechanisms to another. People who have managed to go through these transitions successfully have often used resilience strategies. One resilience strategy is to find sources of strength through media and popular culture. Find a song that has helped you in the past to find peace or transcendence or give you courage. Share the song with the group.

2. The Young and Well (YAW) Cooperative Research Centre is a newly established Australian research centre dedicated to advancing the mental health and wellbeing of young people. Find out what YAW's vision is for young people and identify the types of problems being addressed through research being undertaken by YAW partners.

Websites

Australian Infant, Child, Adolescent and Family Mental Health Association Ltd (AICAFMHA): **www.aicafmha.net.au**
Children of Parents with a Mental Illness (COPMI): **www.copmi.net.au**
Headspace: **www.headspace.org.au**
Orygen Youth Health: **www.oyh.org.au**
Young and Well Cooperative Research Centre: **www.yawcrc.org.au**
Youth Mental Health First Aid Course: **www.mhfa.com.au**

Text links

Chapters 4, 9, 13 and 24 in Elder R, Evans K, Nizette D 2013 Psychiatric and mental health nursing, 3rd edn. Elsevier, Sydney

References

Burns J, Davenport T, Durkin L, Luscombe G, Hickie I 2010 The internet as a setting for mental health service utilisation by young people. Medical Journal of Australia 192(11): S22–S26

McAllister M, Zimmer-Gembeck M, Moyle W, Billett S 2008 Working effectively with clients who self-injure using a solution focused approach. Journal of International Emergency Nursing 16:272–279

Rasmussen P, Henderson A, Muir-Cochrane E 2012 An analysis of the work of child and adolescent mental health nurses in an inpatient unit in Australia. Journal of Psychiatric and Mental Health Nursing 19(4):374–377

A final word

Rachel states:

> I think that nurses look at the whole person and I think that acting early is going to make a positive difference. Child and youth mental health is a really exciting field to work in. It offers lots of personal insights and because you see positive outcomes, it's really, really rewarding.

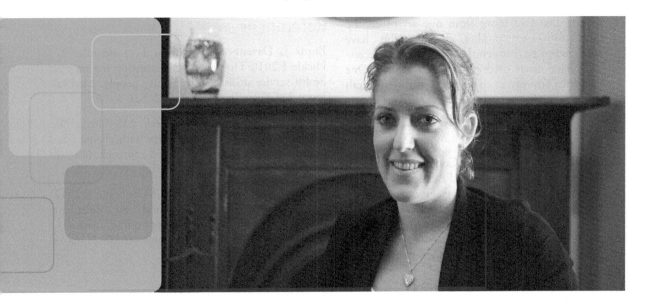

Nadine's story: Having a parent with a mental illness

Introduction

Nadine is a young woman whose mother has been living with early-onset dementia for close to 10 years, since she was in her early 50s. Nadine tells how dementia has affected her mother, including relationships inside the family and with friends. Nadine's mother experiences difficulties in most aspects of her life and is dependent on others for all activities of daily living. But having those needs met, and being treated kindly and with respect, has been an ongoing challenge. Nadine talks about what she wishes for other families who are affected by dementia and what nurses could be doing to make a real difference.

Quick facts

Dementia is not a normal part of the ageing process. And, as in Nadine's experience, it doesn't occur exclusively in older people.

View Nadine's story on evolve
http://evolve.elsevier.com/AU/
Nizette/stories/

Videos

1. Our family and dementia
2. Identity of a carer
3. Don't talk to me, talk to mum

Reflection

1. Keep in mind Nadine's message that people with dementia and their families are individuals: 'They're not "dementias"'. How would you like to be treated if you were in a nursing home?
2. Nadine talks about finding meaning in the experience. Finding meaning is an important asset for a carer's wellbeing. Reflect on how Nadine has coped throughout this experience.

Inquiry

1. As you listen to Nadine's retelling of the impact that dementia is having on her family relationships, make a note of the phases that occurred with her mother's experience, noting the impact that changes had on her identity, relationships and being in the world.
2. Allport's (1954) theory of discrimination and prejudice suggests that the first step in dehumanising someone is to talk about them rather than to them. **Brainstorming activity:** Reflect

Language practices that support identity and include the person	Language practices that strip away identity and exclude the person

on interactions between nurse and client that you have observed in the workplace or in the media and complete the table above.

Action

1. How could you learn about the person's story and how might this change your interpretation and reaction to the complex behaviours associated with dementia?
2. Create a memory board indicating what you want your carers to know about you when *you* go to a nursing home.
3. Exploring Seligman's PERMA framework, what aspects of Nadine's story helped to build her resilience?

Websites

For the dementia collaborative research centres, start here:

Dementia Collaborative Research Centres: **www.dementia.unsw.edu.au**
Dementia Friendly Environments: **www.health.vic.gov.au/dementia/strategies/home-like-environment-checklist.htm**
For a checklist on creating home-like environments in the unit where you work, start here:
Children of People with Mental Illness: **www.copmi.net.au**
Home-like Environment Checklist: **www.health.vic.gov.au/dementia/strategies/home-like-environment-checklist.htm**

Text links

Chapters 4, 13 and 14 in Elder R, Evans K, Nizette D 2013 Psychiatric and mental health nursing, 3rd edn. Elsevier, Sydney

References

Allport G 1954 The nature of prejudice. Doubleday/Anchor, New York

Moyle W 2009 Mental disorders in the aged. In Elder R, Evans K, Nizette D Psychiatric and mental health nursing. Elsevier, Sydney

Moyle W, Kellett U, Ballantyne A, Gracia N 2011 Dementia and loneliness: an Australian perspective. Journal of Clinical Nursing 20(9–10):1445–1453

Wei Z, Cooke M, Moyle W, Creedy D 2010 Health education needs of family caregivers supporting an adolescent relative with schizophrenia or a mood disorder in Taiwan. Archives of Psychiatric Nursing 24(6):418–428

A final word

Nadine is a daughter who loves her mother and has an experience that unfortunately too many people who are children of parents with mental illness (COPMI) share: distress, uncertainty and being powerless to change what's happened. But if we as students of nursing listen to her message, we begin to really understand that mental disorder doesn't just affect the individual: it affects families too. If we are to be effective in facilitating transition to wellbeing, acceptance and recovery, then families need to be our partners in care.

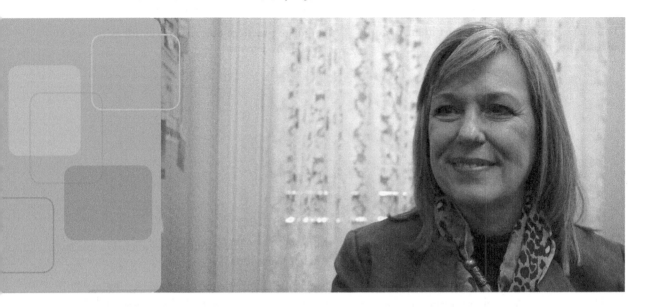

Tara's story: Humanising dementia care

Introduction

Tara Quirke is an RN with qualifications in mental health nursing and gerontology. She has experience working as a nurse in nursing homes and as a manager. She currently works as an aged care assessor, visiting residential care settings to oversee the implementation of Australian Aged Care Standards and the Aged Care Act (1997).

Quick facts

Dementia is a broad term used to describe a large range of illnesses that cause progressive decline in a person's functioning, including loss of memory and ability to think and learn. There are numerous types of dementia, including Alzheimer's, Parkinson's disease, Pick's disease and frontotemporal dementia. Mental health problems and disabilities often come hand in hand with dementia, including psychosis, anxiety, depression, aggression, loneliness and relationship disturbance.

View Tara's story on evolve
http://evolve.elsevier.com/AU/
Nizette/stories/

Videos

1. All behaviour has meaning
2. Philosophy of dementia care
3. Looking differently at aged care

Reflection

1. Person-centred care is tailored around a person's likes and dislikes.
2. Working with older people is interesting and enriching. When you take the time to get to know the person, where they've come from, what changes they've seen, what lessons they've learned, what makes them happy, what makes them sad, you will understand the secret power of nursing. It's really all about learning to be truly human. How do you hope that nursing will impact on your growth as a person?

Inquiry

1. Why do you think so many people tend to reach for medications as an intervention to manage problems? What are the dangers in using medications as the first action, or only intervention, in

the context of old age? What medications are of use and for what conditions? What principles should guide their use?

2. What does Tara suggest may help nurses and other caregivers to look beyond the surface behaviours and emotional expressions to enhance the person's capacity to live a fully human, and humanising, life?

3. Tara makes a point about the dominance of control mechanisms, such as the use of restraints and medication, in caring for people with dementia. Investigate alternative models of care.

Action

1. What is the benefit of the metaphor 'nurse as investigator' in this care-giving context? How does it compare with the metaphor 'nurse as custodian'?

2. Think of all the behaviours of a 'caretaker' (who cleans, and completes tasks to provide hygienic standards) and compare these with the behaviours of an 'investigator' (who tracks down clues, and is alert to all data, to find the source of problems).

3. How could the metaphor 'nurse as investigator' be applied to nursing work in this context?

Activities

1. Undertake an internet search to find five behavioural and psychological symptoms of dementia (BPSD). What are some main questions to explore about BPSD?

2. Find best-practice guidelines on these issues. In your group, discuss best practice in responding to each of these symptoms.

3. Tara mentions the Eden Alternative. Investigate this and other innovations such as:

- Gentlecare™
- digital storytelling.

Websites

For information on Australian aged care services, start here:

Australian Ageing Agenda: **www.australianageing agenda.com.au**

Department of Health and Ageing: **http:// agedcareaustralia.gov.au**

Eden in Oz & NZ: **www.edeninoznz.com.au/ html/s01_home/home.asp**

Gentlecare: **www.toronto.ca/ltc/pdf/gentlecare_ bro.pdf**

University of Wollongong: **www.uow.edu.au/ crearts/news/UOW045396.html**

Text links

Chapters 2, 8, 9 and 14 in Elder R, Evans K, Nizette D 2013 Psychiatric and mental health nursing, 3rd edn. Elsevier, Sydney

References

Holm A, Lepp M, Ringsberg K 2005 Dementia: involving patients in storytelling—a caring intervention. A pilot study. Journal of Clinical Nursing 14(2):256–263

Kellett U, Moyle W, McAllister M, King C, Gallagher F 2010 Life stories and biography: a means of connecting family and staff to people with dementia. Journal of Clinical Nursing 19(11–12):1707–1715

A final word

Tara has a vision for Australia that all people with dementia will be cared for in a truly person-centred way. Tara, as a highly experienced dementia-care specialist, is an outspoken and influential activist. She is also someone who had the privilege of living with and caring for her father who had dementia until he died one evening, with his favourite music playing and his faithful old cat asleep on his lap.

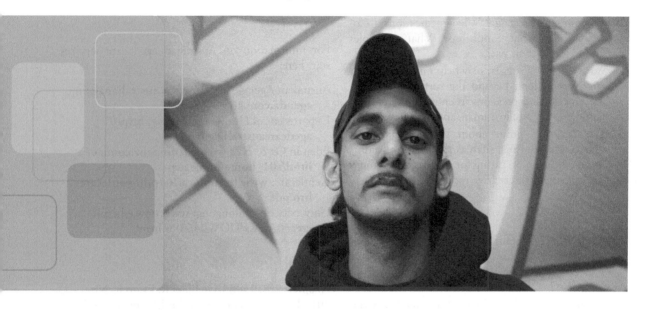

Jeremy's story: Beliefs and perceptions

Introduction

Jeremy is a young man who is experiencing psychotic phenomena in the context of significant substance abuse and associated criminal behaviour. Jeremy is accessing treatment with Toby at his 'clinic without walls'.

View Jeremy's story on evolve
http://evolve.elsevier.com/AU/
Nizette/stories/

Videos

1. Symptoms are different for everybody
2. When you ask me that, it gets me somewhere
3. Medication can be a short-term crutch

Reflection

1. Jeremy is very focused on the impact of religion on his life—both positive and negative—and this is reflected in how his symptoms are experienced. Consider how this might make him feel and how it might impact on your responses to him. What aspects of Jeremy's story do you feel empathy with?

2. Toby addresses the common and challenging issue facing consumers with psychosis and that is treatment adherence. How does Toby raise the issue of balancing the therapeutic effect of medication with listening to Jeremy's concerns?

3. One of the particular skills of nurses working with people with psychosis is being able to determine whether their thoughts are within the range of 'normal' or are delusional. Notice how Toby drills down on the beliefs Jeremy has about reading people's minds.

Inquiry

1. How can you tell that Toby is using active listening with Jeremy?
2. What is the mental health nurse's role in relation to medication?
3. Investigate the psychological effects of the illicit substances that Jeremy refers to in the interview. How does substance use impact on mental health?

Action

1. Suggested assignment: a written report entitled 'When is a clinician therapeutic?'
2. Discuss some common symptoms that people with psychosis experience and match these to any Jeremy may display in the interview.

3. Listen to the interview. How does Toby deliver important psycho education to Jeremy?

4. Access a Mental State Examination tool and in pairs, as you watch the video, try to complete the examination with a particular focus on affect, content of thought and form of thought. Share your findings with the group.

Websites

Early Psychosis Prevention and Intervention Centre: **www.eppic.org.au**

GROW Australia: **www.grow.net.au**

Mental Illness fellowship of Australia Inc.: **www.mifa.org.au**

SANE Australia: **www.sane.org**

Suicide Prevention Australia: **http://suicide preventionaust.org**

Text links

Chapters 5, 11, 15, 16, 24 and 26 in Elder R, Evans K, Nizette D 2013 Psychiatric and mental health nursing, 3rd edn. Elsevier, Sydney

References

Dunn SV, Cashin AJ, Buckley T, Newman C 2010 Nurse practitioner prescribing practice in Australia. Journal of the American Academy of Nurse Practitioners 22(3):150–155

Gardiner A, Hase S, Gardner G, Dunn SV, Carryer J 2008 Nurse practitioner competence and capability. Journal of Clinical Nursing 17:250–258

Gray R, White J, Schulz M, Abderhalden C 2010 Enhancing medication adherence in people with schizophrenia: an international programme of research. International Journal of Mental Health Nursing 19(1):36–44

Lorem FG, Hem MH 2012 Attuned understanding and psychotic suffering: a qualitative study of health-care professionals' experiences in communicating and interacting with patients. International Journal of Mental Health Nursing 21(2):114–122

A final word

Jeremy has friends, a girlfriend and a positive sense of self and is developing a trusting relationship with his gentle, empathic and concerned case manager. Jeremy engages honestly with Toby because he trusts him. And Toby shows us that it is possible to probe the depth and impact of symptoms of psychosis without being intrusive, pushy or rude. Psychosis is a major mental disorder that disrupts people's lives, but with support and careful management people can live happy and productive lives.

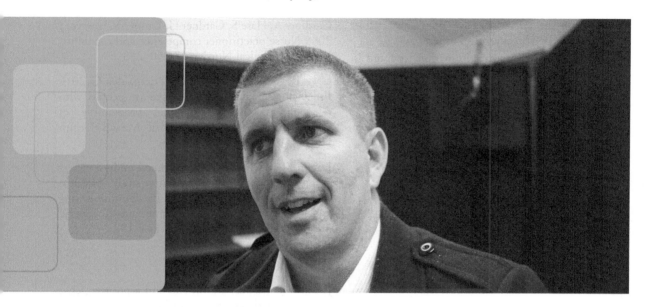

Toby's story: Providing an accessible service

Introduction

Toby is a mental health nurse working as a nurse practitioner in autonomous practice. He works with colleagues providing mental healthcare, primarily to young people from vulnerable groups. He describes the charity he has established, where he works in settings he describes as a 'clinic without walls'. Many people using this service have struggled to get help from other health services and to be given the time to tell their story. Toby talks about his practice and the importance of getting the whole picture.

 View Toby's story on evolve
http://evolve.elsevier.com/AU/
Nizette/stories/

Videos

1. A clinic without walls
2. Getting the whole picture

Reflection

1. When else have you heard the term 'without walls' or 'without borders'? What opportunities does a service without walls offer? How do these services support people in recovery?
2. With reference to Jeremy's story, what parts of Jeremy's picture can you put together? If you were in Toby's shoes, what aspects of Jeremy's story would you be particularly interested in?
3. Listen to Toby's interview with Jeremy and identify the therapeutic communication skills used and when they are used. Comment on one part of the interview that you think was done well and why you chose that part.

Inquiry

1. How are the aims of mental health nursing reflected in Toby's comment about trying to get the whole picture (when working with consumers)? What do mental health nursing theorists say about this? (Consider the theorists Hildegard Peplau, Gene Watson and Imogen King.)
2. Toby uses a timeline to work with Jeremy. What can timelines be used for?

Action

1. Make a list of the mental health services available/accessible in your area. Identify those that could be defined as services 'without walls'.

2. If you were a consumer, would you be able to access a range of services 'seamlessly'?

Websites

Early Psychosis Prevention and Intervention Centre: **www.eppic.org.au**

GROW Australia: **www.grow.net.au**

Mental Illness Fellowship of Australia Inc.: **www.mifa.org.au**

SANE Australia: **www.sane.org**

Suicide Prevention Australia: **http://suicide preventionaust.org**

Text links

Chapters 1, 5, 6, 8, 23 and 25 in Elder R, Evans K, Nizette D 2013 Psychiatric and mental health nursing, 3rd edn. Elsevier, Sydney

References

Gray R, White J, Schulz M, Abderhalden C 2010 Enhancing medication adherence in people with schizophrenia: an international programme of research. International Journal of Mental Health Nursing 19(1):36–44

Van Meijel B, Van Der Gaag M, Sylvain R, Grypdonck M 2004 Recognition of early warning signs in patients with schizophrenia: a review of the literature. International Journal of Mental Health Nursing 13(2):107–116

A final word

Toby states:

> The first thing that I would do is acknowledge that medication is only ever part of the story. I place the young person at the centre of their own care, acknowledging their right to choose.

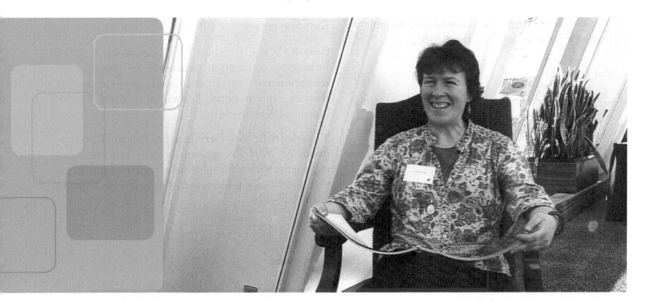

Lorraine's story: A creative consumer advocate

Introduction

Lorraine Nicholson is author and illustrator of the book *The Journey Home*, which chronicles her experience with and emergence from depression into recovery. Key themes: recovery; hope.

View Lorraine's story on evolve
http://evolve.elsevier.com/AU/
Nizette/stories/

Video used with permission of the Scottish Recovery Network.

Reflection

1. Listen to Lorraine and focus on the content and style of her artistic work. Lorraine comments that her recovery was not just about becoming free of symptoms of depression, but also about finding colour again. This encapsulates the notion that mental health is not just the absence of illness, but is a positive state, one where people can flourish.

2. Go to the Hands on Scotland website to find out what is meant by a 'flourishing state'.

3. What does Seligman's concept of PERMA stand for? How can these components be enacted to promote recovery?

4. How do you think professional nurses can integrate concepts of flourishing, so that work with individuals and productive workplaces can become more about wellbeing and not just illness-care?

5. Lorraine mentions that sometimes deeply engaging in an inspiring poem can become a turning point for a person. Listen to (or read) Lorraine's poem *Seeing the light in me*. Imagine that Lorraine has written this poem about you when you were her nurse.

6. How do you feel after reading this poem?

7. What do you think Lorraine means by her plea for nurses to 'see the light'?

8. What does Lorraine mean by her protest about 'being packaged and dehumanised', and what insights do you have about the poem?

9. What are the key principles for nurses seeking to encourage clients to participate in their health management?

10. What is Lorraine's personal meaning of recovery? How is it different from, or the same as, other experiences you have heard in other stories?

Inquiry

1. In her poem *Unashamed*, Lorraine speaks about 'internalised stigma' and acceptance of self

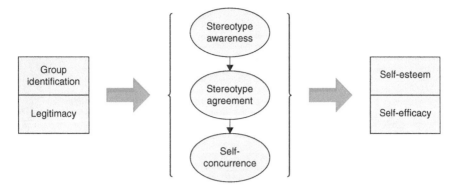

Figure 5 The Theoretical Model of Self Stigma
source: Amy C. Watson, Patrick Corrigan, Jonathon E. Larson, Molly Sells, Self-Stigma in People With Mental Illness, Schizophrenia Bulletin, (2007) 33 (6):1312-1318, by permission of Oxford University Press, http://schizophreniabulletin. oxfordjournals.org/content/33/6/1312.full

emerging from darkness. Investigate the concept of internalised stigma. The articles by Ritscher, Ottingham and Grajales, 'Internalized stigma of mental illness: psychometric properties of a new measure' (at **www.sciencedirect.com/science/article/pii/ S0165178103002075**) and by Watson et al (at **http://schizophreniabulletin.oxfordjournals. org/content/33/6/1312.full**) are a starting point from which to explore the literature on internalised stigma. What strategies can you identify and use in your role as a nurse to help people to address internalised stigma?

2. Using Watson et al's Theoretical Model of Self Stigma (see Figure 5), write a short article on how stigma impacts on self-esteem and self-acceptance.

Action

1. Meet with a person working in a peer support worker role. Think about how the system has adapted to consumers sharing their lived experience. Develop a role description (if you can) and propose a staffing profile for a public health service. (For example, what staff/roles do you need in a public mental health service, and what would they do?) It might be helpful to get the perspective of a consumer or peer support worker for this activity.

2. Lorraine talks about using her book as a journal of her experiences. Journaling has been used to facilitate reflection on practice in nursing. Use the tips in the references below and keep a journal (a book or Word file) of your practice.

3. Search through the following resources or other artworks and select a piece that you think could provide an inspiring message and increase the belief and hope that recovery is possible:

- poems produced by Lorraine Nicholson, Sandy Jeffs and others
- virtual art galleries such as those at **http:// eliminatethestigma.wordpress.com/ art-gallery** and **www.bethlemgallery.com/ Bethlem_Gallery/Welcome.html**
- song lyrics by singers such as Nirvana, the Good Charlotte or Don Maclean.

Text links

Chapters 2, 16, 24 and 25 in Elder R, Evans K, Nizette D 2013 Psychiatric and mental health nursing, 3rd edn. Elsevier, Sydney

Websites

Beyond Blue: **www.beyondblue.org.au/index.aspx**
Black Dog Institute: **www.blackdoginstitute.org.au**
Hands on Scotland: **www.handsonscotland.co.uk**

References

Billings D 2006 Journaling: a strategy for developing reflective practitioners. The Journal of Continuing Education in Nursing 37(3):104–105

Stickley T, Hui A, 2012 Arts in-reach: taking 'bricks off shoulders' in adult mental health inpatient care. Journal of Psychiatric and Mental Health Nursing 19(5):402–409

Wagner AL 2002 Nursing students' development of caring self through reflective practice. In Freshwater D Therapeutic nursing: improving patient care through self-awareness and reflection. Sage, London, pp 121–130

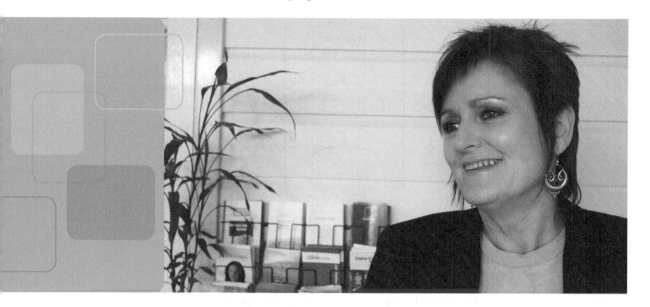

Christine's story: Primary mental healthcare

Introduction

Christine Palmer is a Credentialed Mental Health Nurse who works in private practice. A significant amount of her work is provided under the Commonwealth government's Mental Health Nurse Incentive Program. Under this program Christine works collaboratively with general practitioners and private psychiatrists to provide collaborative primary mental healthcare.

 View Christine's story on evolve
http://evolve.elsevier.com/AU/
Nizette/stories/

Videos

1. About the program
2. The therapeutic relationship

Reflection

1. Listen to Christine's comments on how she establishes and maintains a therapeutic relationship with a client.
2. An important element of Christine's practice is clinical supervision. What exactly is clinical supervision, and how does it differ from employee management?

Inquiry

A core aspect of contemporary mental health nursing is the recovery model. It is important that you understand what this means and can distinguish recovery models from curative and rehabilitation approaches. Chapter 2 in Elder, Evans and Nizette (2013) provides an important foundation.

Action

Use the therapeutic appraisal tool in Table 2 to identify key aspects of Christine's intended approaches that you could develop in your own practice.

Websites

Australian College of Mental Health Nurses: **www.achmn.org**
Community Mental Health Australia: **www.cmha.org.au/projects.html**
Medicare Australia: **www.medicareaustralia.gov.au/provider/incentives/mhnip/index.jsp**
National Mental Health Development Unit: **www.nmhdu.org.uk/our-work/mhep/delivering-race-equality/dre-recovery**

Table 2 Therapeutic appraisal

Responsiveness	Yes/no
Attends to the person (not just the problem)	
Explores the person's perspective of what's happened	
Explores what the person would like to do/be	
Varies affect expression and nonverbal responses (posture, eye contact, smiles, head nods) according to the person's communication	
Matches mood	
Responds to questions appropriately	
Other	
Warm engagement	
Expresses concern and caring in relevant, appropriate ways	
Emotional expression by the person is accepted	
Invites client to engage in an ongoing therapeutic conversation	
Other	
Identifying goals for change through	
Supporting, validating, motivating change	
Seeking feedback on own actions	
General comments and suggestions	

Text links

Chapters 1, 2, 21, 23 and 25 in Elder R, Evans K, Nizette D 2013 Psychiatric and mental health nursing, 3rd edn. Elsevier, Sydney

References

ACMHN statement on clinical supervision. Available at **www.acmhn.org/career-resources/clinical-supervision.html**

Gardner A 2010 Therapeutic friendliness and the development of therapeutic leverage by mental health nurses in community rehabilitation settings. Contemporary Nurse 34(2):140–148

A final word

Professional mental health nurses have the knowledge as well as the know-how, the personal qualities to be able to connect with clients on a human and yet caring level, and the insight to be able to seek external support to process, learn from and debrief challenging issues.

Christine states:

Since I've been working in primary mental health-care, these last three and a half years, I've been much more conscious of the change in focus in my practice, and I see that there's potential for all mental health nurses, regardless of the context of your work. So whether you work in an in-patient unit or in a community service or a rehabilitation unit, that focus needs to be on building people's strength and their resilience, so that it's not about responding or reacting to exacerbation of illness but actually working with people towards their recovery and building their strengths so they're less likely to have another exacerbation of their condition … That they actually have the capacity to live meaningful lives, and they're able to get on and do that.

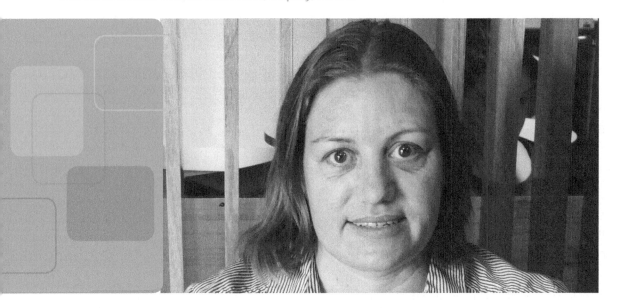

Catherine's story: Reframing personality disorder

Introduction

Catherine has a diagnosis of borderline personality disorder and has endured significant trauma both in her early life and unfortunately in her journey throughout the mental health system. For people with the diagnosis of personality disorder, this is not an uncommon experience. But what makes Catherine's story stand out is that she can articulate her vulnerabilities (and these are ongoing), can channel and divert stressors so that they are less intrusive and pervasive, and is making a positive contribution to the world by being an active consumer representative and advocate.

 View Catherine's story on evolve
http://evolve.elsevier.com/AU/
Nizette/stories/

Reflection

1. As you listen to Catherine's story, make a timeline of her journey. Identify key issues that became (a) obstacles to and (b) facilitators of health and wellbeing.
2. Make a two-column table. In one column list the common issues for people with BPD and in the other list potential outcomes if better therapy and standards of care were available.
3. What do you think are the keys to Catherine's ongoing recovery?
4. Self-harm is a very common behaviour that can be used as a coping mechanism—useful in the short term, but damaging in the long term. Self-harm is really the absence of self-care. As a beginning clinician you will need to put boundaries around any coping mechanisms that you have used in the past and make sure that these do not impact on the therapeutic relationship. Being self-aware helps you to not inadvertently slip into using unconscious coping mechanisms. Remind yourself about unconscious coping mechanisms by reviewing Chapter 8 in Elder, Evans and Nizette (2013).

Inquiry

1. Go to the web page of SPECTRUM (the personality disorder service for Victoria; see the website listing below) and read about borderline personality disorder so that you have an understanding of its clinical picture.
2. Listen to Catherine's conversation and note down any symptoms and experiences that she reports that appear to fit this clinical picture of borderline personality disorder.

Action

Seek out resources that you can use in your professional practice to educate consumers, carers, school teachers and other clinicians about self-injury and about ways of being therapeutic. Make sure that the information is from reliable, reputable sources, backed up with trustworthy evidence, and is unlikely to trigger episodes of trauma or harm to the reader. Use the websites below as a good place to start your search.

Websites

Centre for Suicide Prevention Studies: **www. suicidepreventionstudies.com**
Project Air Strategy for Personality Disorders: **http://ihmri.uow.edu.au/projectairstrategy/ index.html**
SBS Secrets of the Human Body: **www.sbs.com.au/ shows/secretsofthehumanbody/tab-listings/ page/i/4/h/The-Silent-Epidemic**
Spectrum Personality Disorder Service for VIC: **www.spectrumbpd.com.au**

Text links

Chapters 8, 10, 17 and 24 in Elder R, Evans K, Nizette D 2013 Psychiatric and mental health nursing, 3rd edn. Elsevier, Sydney

References

Clarkin J 2006 Conceptualization and treatment of personality disorders. Psychotherapy Research 16(1):1–11

McAllister M 2003 Multiple meanings of self-harm: a critical review. International Journal of Mental Health Nursing 12(3):177–185

McAllister M, Zimmer-Gembeck M, Moyle W, Billett S 2008 Working effectively with clients who self-injure using a solution-focused approach. Journal of International Emergency Nursing 16:272–279

Martin G, Hasking P, Swannell S, McAllister M 2010 Seeking solutions to self-injury: a guide for parents and families. Centre for Suicide Prevention Studies, University of Queensland. Available at **www. suicidepreventionstudies.com**

A final word

Catherine states:

> No one chooses to have a personality disorder, no one chooses to be addicted to self-harming, no one chooses to have extreme emotions, but this has happened to them. This is something that has happened to them and they're the ones suffering and that's where the compassion needs to come in.

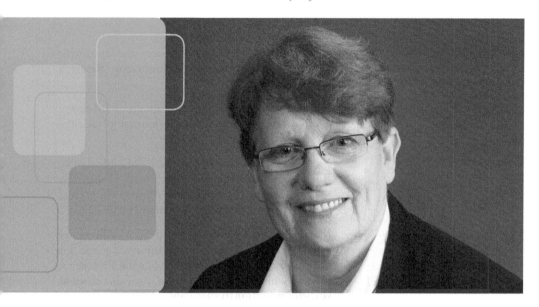

Louise's story: On conversational models

Introduction

Throughout this podcast you will hear Louise O'Brien, Professor of Nursing and a Credentialed Mental Health Nurse who works in private practice with clients who have been diagnosed with personality disorder, discuss why she enjoys the challenge of working with this client group.

 View Louise's story on evolve
http://evolve.elsevier.com/AU/
Nizette/stories/

Reflection

1. Louise emphasises that to be an effective therapist nurses need ego competencies themselves. Identify your personal ego strengths.
2. What does Louise caution that nurses need to be aware of in ensuring that they remain therapeutic?
3. Nurses can be very effective in the short term. Louise notes that beginning nurses working in acute or short-term settings can support consumers with gross ego dysfunction and extreme behaviours by providing a holding environment. How could your interpersonal skills be used to provide a holding environment for consumers who are very distressed?
4. What is the difference between psychological splitting and interpersonal splitting?
5. Reflect on Louise's closing comments. Reflect on a time when your feelings were validated. How can you use similar validation with clients, regardless of the time you have available to spend with them?
6. How do you intend to 'reject the rejecting language' that you are likely to encounter from misguided or ill-informed colleagues?

Inquiry

A person with borderline personality disorder has a disturbance of self. One way to understand this is through thinking about the ego and the strength of the ego.

Strayhorn (1989, in Stuart & Laraia, 1998) identified the following skills that all children need to become competent adults:

- establishing closeness and trusting relationships
- handling separation and independent decision making
- negotiating joint decisions and interpersonal conflict

- dealing with frustration and unfavourable events
- celebrating good feelings and experiencing pleasure
- relaxing and playing
- cognitive processing through words, symbols and images
- establishing an adaptive sense of direction and purpose.

1. Nurses can support the person's ego functioning by being a positive role model. Louise talks about how she supports a person's ego function. From what Louise says, identify things that she does to support a person's ego functioning.
2. Louise uses a conversational model in her work with consumers experiencing borderline personality disorder. This is a powerful way to support ego strength, by modelling and teaching ways of relating competently. Use the skills list above to explore what ego strengths can be developed in a therapeutic conversation. Identify similarities with a strengths model.
3. What do all effective therapies for borderline personality disorder have in common? (Emphasise the holding environment, acceptance and change.)
4. Identify the difference between psychological splitting and interpersonal splitting.
5. Louise makes the point that boundaries define what it is you do as a nurse and what you don't do and how you ensure that you don't overstep the mark. Louise states: 'it's not the client's job to actually manage the boundary; it's the staff's job.' What does Louise say about boundaries and people with borderline personality disorder? (For more about boundaries, see Elder, Evans & Nizette, 2013.) Consider also how Christine Palmer talks about boundaries working autonomously in the primary care setting.
6. Louise lists a lot of different components for the system to be therapeutic. The clinical setting can have a therapeutic system in place to ensure the environment remains therapeutic. Make a list of all the components that Louise mentions as important to supporting this productive system.
7. Outline strategies that the system has in place to support the clinician and the consumer.

Action

1. Explore the literature on the ego competency model to identify other ways that nurses can support someone to develop a more positive sense of self.

2. Talk to people and make notes on the idea of the 'therapeutic use of self'. Discuss these ideas in a tutorial group or with colleagues.
3. Louise asserts that healthcare teams need to enact a model of care for people with personality disorders and to stop responding in unplanned, reactive, emotional and stigmatising ways. Make a memorable diagram or mnemonic to help you and your colleagues facilitate better nursing care for people with this experience.

Websites

BPD Central: **www.bpdcentral.com**
Reachout: **http://au.reachout.com**
SANE Australia: **www.sane.org/information/ factsheets-podcasts/160-borderline- personality-disorder**
Spectrum: **www.spectrumbpd.com.au**

Text links

Chapters 1, 17 and 25 in Elder R, Evans K, Nizette D 2013 Psychiatric and mental health nursing, 3rd edn. Elsevier, Sydney

Reference

Stuart GW, Laraia MT 1998 Principles and practice of psychiatric nursing, 6th edn. Mosby, St Louis

A final word

Reflect on Louise O'Brien's closing words and, with a highlighter pen, identify keywords that you would want others to remember:

> Even in short, brief contact with those clients. Even if you were a nurse working in [an] accident [and] emergency department who sees people coming in with having self-harmed. Those brief encounters, if they are compassionate and validating for the person and recognise that you know that they must have been distressed when this was happening, and they weren't being difficult and just there to make your life difficult, I think in that kind of encounter, you can make a difference.

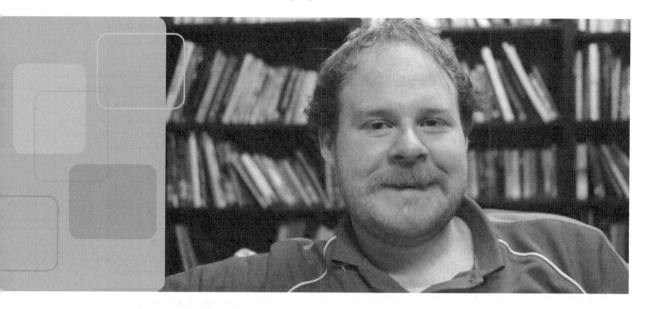

Jarrad's story: Containing fear

Introduction

Jarrad is a young man who has an anxiety disorder that affects him in profound ways. It first developed in his middle school years and his daily struggles surround managing intrusive thoughts, controlling the physical effects of anxiety on his whole bodily system and continuing to be sociable when he feels frightened of what could happen in an uncontrolled social setting.

 View Jarrad's story on evolve
http://evolve.elsevier.com/AU/
Nizette/stories/

Videos

1. Anxiety just snowballs
2. A traumatic experience
3. Easing into treatment

Reflection

1. While it is important to attend to a person's nonverbal communication, mental health nurses appreciate that what a person is displaying outwardly may not always correspond with what they are experiencing inwardly. Discuss this notion after observing Jarrad's affect and listening to what he says he experiences in relation to his anxiety.
2. What lesson have you learned about empathy from this exercise?
3. Students of mental health don't need to be 'experts' to be helpful. Jarrad describes that there are fewer 'us and them' boundaries between him and nursing students, who he feels are more his contemporaries rather than his therapists. What was the beneficial role of nursing students in Jarrad's journey? Reflect on times that you have been able to help without taking an 'expert' stance. What can you take from this experience of helping into your role as expert?

Inquiry

1. What did Toby say had helped Jarrad? What therapeutic models relate most closely to this?
2. Investigate what early intervention might mean in relation to managing anxiety.
3. 'Reframing' is a concept used in anxiety management. What is it and what does it involve? Can you find some examples?

4. Jarrad talks about how the experience of stress makes his anxiety worse. What is the physiological relationship between the two?

Action

1. Use the ABC model of listening to make a concerted effort to attend to the content of what Jarrad is saying during the interview.
2. As you listen to Jarrad's responses to the interviewer, make a note of the range of thoughts that are part of the picture of his anxiety and stress.
3. Jarrad talks about keeping himself in the moment and distracting himself by focusing on the knowledge he now has about the physiological effects of anxiety. Prepare an overview of the physiological processes associated with anxiety, in terms that you would use to describe them to a client.
4. Develop a mindfulness exercise and conduct it with your tutorial group.

Websites

Anxiety Recovery Centre Victoria: **www.arcvic. org.au**

Beyond Blue: **www.beyondblue.org.au/index. aspx?link_id=90**

Mindfulness: **www.mindfulness.org.au/links. html**

Reachout: **http://au.reachout.com/find/articles/ anxiety**

SANE Australia: **www.sane.org/information/ factsheets-podcasts/158-anxiety-disorders**

Text links

Chapters 1, 17, 18 and 25 in Elder R, Evans K, Nizette D 2013 Psychiatric and mental health nursing, 3rd edn. Elsevier, Sydney

References

Kerr N 1990 The ego competency model of psychiatric nursing: theoretical overview and clinical application. Perspectives in Psychiatric Care 26(1):13–24

Linehan M 1995 Understanding borderline personality disorder: the dialectical approach. Program Manual. Guilford Press, New York

A final word

Anxiety, as Jarrad helps us to see, is not always merely a minor annoyance in a person's life. When it is severe enough to become a disorder, it is a serious mental illness that can suddenly make its presence felt, or sneak up insidiously. For Jarrad, it seems, one year he was living a care-free and happy life and the next he was frozen with fear, unable to control intrusive and destructive thoughts. Extreme anxiety can take away people's sense of peace. It can destroy lives. But Jarrad has—through determination, guidance and support—learned to take back control, and his is an inspirational story of practice and acceptance.

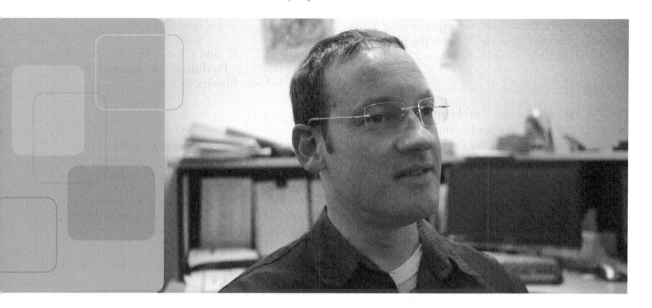

Todd's story: Consultation liaison

Introduction

Todd works as a psychiatric consultation liaison nurse and responds to requests for mental health expertise from general medical and surgical units of a large hospital. His work involves providing support, assessment, diagnosis or treatment for clients with physical health problems who are experiencing emotional distress. In this interview, Todd focuses particularly on clients who have a respiratory disorder and experience anxiety.

View Todd's story on evolve
http://evolve.elsevier.com/AU/
Nizette/stories/

Videos

1. A day in the life
2. Assessing anxiety
3. What you can do

Reflection

1. Todd is a specialist mental health nurse and has the skills to differentiate between the different types of anxiety. What could you do to help someone through distress and anxiety, and when would you know to refer the person to someone like Todd?
2. Todd raises the image of birds startling each other off the tree—responding instinctively to each other. How can you overcome the tendency to be influenced by someone else's anxiety and be the bird that stays on the branch? What strategies will help you to do this?

Inquiry

1. As you can hear on listening to Todd's account, managing a person's anxiety is a prominent part of Todd's practice. What are the major health conditions that Todd discusses?
2. Read Chapter 18 in Elder, Evans and Nizette (2013) to identify the major types of anxiety disorders.

Action

Everyone gets anxious from time to time. In fact, anxiety performs a valuable early-warning signal that something is not right or safe either inside or outside our body. It is common to feel anxiety when faced with something strange or new, or when anticipating change and we don't know whether it will be good or bad. A small amount of anxiety improves performance and motivates us to take action. However, when anxiety interferes with daily living and goal achievement and is present to the extent that it causes uncomfortable or even frightening feelings, it may be defined as a disorder. Anxiety is a very common experience for all people utilising healthcare. Hospitals are strange environments, where people's needs are not always fully met. Having health investigations may increase their anticipation and worry.

Differentiate between 'normal' anxiety and anxiety disorders.

Websites

AIHW Comorbidity of Mental Disorders and Physical Conditions, 2007 (released 2012): **www.aihw.gov.au/publication-detail/?id=10737421146**

Australian Depression & Anxiety Alliance: **www.adaaa.com.au**

Clinical Guidelines for the Physical Care of Mental Health Consumers: **www.psychiatry.uwa.edu.au/research/community-culture/physical-care-clinical-guidelines**

Policy document—Physical Health Care of Mental Health Consumers: **www.health.nsw.gov.au/policies/gl/2009/GL2009_007.html**

Reachout: **www.reachout.com** (contains a podcast of a woman's experience with anxiety; as well as a strategy called 'the broken record', which is helpful in interrupting the broken record that keeps looping in your head)

Text links

Chapters 1, 18 and 25 in Elder R, Evans K, Nizette D 2013 Psychiatric and mental health nursing, 3rd edn. Elsevier, Sydney

Reference

Jorm A, Morgan A, Wright A 2010 Actions that young people can take to prevent depression, anxiety and psychosis: beliefs of health professionals and young people. Journal of Affective Disorders 126(1):278–281

A final word

Todd's advanced nursing practice skills enable him to work in a very challenging and rewarding area, as a consultation liaison nurse—yet one more career-advancing opportunity for those who choose mental health nursing as their specialty.

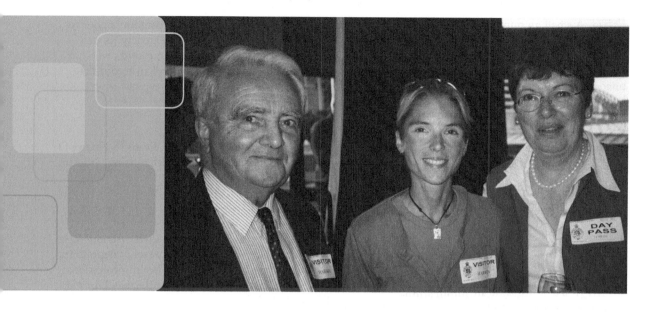

Sonja's story: Finding strengths

Introduction

Sonja St Leon died from anorexia nervosa in 2004. Her parents share her important story, in her memory, to help people understand just how serious anorexia nervosa is.

What you need to know

1. Eating disorders are serious illnesses that have a major negative impact on physical, social, psychological and cognitive health.
2. Standardised mortality rates for eating disorders are 12 times higher than the annual death rate from all causes in females aged 15–24 years; and the mortality rate for suicide in people with eating disorders is the highest of any psychiatric illness.
3. Despite the media focus on celebrities who develop eating disorders, the illnesses are not well understood and are often misrepresented.

View Sonja's story on evolve
http://evolve.elsevier.com/AU/
Nizette/stories/

Reflection

1. Make a table with two columns. In one column, list the self-defeating behaviours and thoughts that are revealed in Sonja's story. In the other column, suggest alternatives that are self-supporting behaviours and thoughts.
2. 'Fat talk' has been said to be a common motif of female culture, particularly in developed countries. Women are encouraged to aspire to an ideal body type, and often say self-disparaging things or communicate with others around this theme. Consider the following commonly heard statement: 'I feel fat today.' This expression is made more commonly by young women than men, and is repeated over and over. But, in fact, the person is actually feeling another emotion, such as worry, guilt or anger. This expression of emotion is effectively covered up by referring instead to an outward physical presence (being fat). So 'fat talk' is actually a metaphor for a feeling. When this notion is identified as a metaphor, it is possible for it to be challenged and replaced. What are some more productive metaphors or statements that you could suggest young women make to help them express their emotions more accurately?

Inquiry

1. Listen to the St Leons retelling what happened to Sonja and the whole family as they watched anorexia nervosa take over their daughter's life. Parents of people with eating disorders often say that their child was the perfect child—well-behaved, perfectionistic, never a worry. The point to note here is that just because a person outwardly presents as competent, happy and in control of their own life, this may not be their internal experience.

2. Holding externalising conversations about how eating disorders affect a person's life, rather than considering the eating disorder as a core part of the person's personality, is an essential therapeutic technique. Search the Dulwich Centre to explore externalising conversations and narrative therapy and to find out:

   • why it may be helpful to put some distance between the person (or self) and the mental health problems

   • how to engage in an externalising conversation

   • what the effects of externalising a problem are

   • how to hold an externalising conversation about 'the eating disorder' with families, clinical colleagues and others.

Action

1. Examine Ancel Keys' (1950) famous Starvation Study (start with this vimeo clip) and find more detail through an online search). This study explains that when starvation syndrome takes hold, the body physiologically becomes driven to meet primal needs and it becomes impossible to engage in more complex neurological functions, such as reasoning.

2. Some clinicians assume that, because of prominent features such as self-preoccupation and anti-social behaviours, anorexia nervosa is a type of personality disorder. How does the information in the Starvation Study challenge this assumption?

3. What components do you need to assess (cognitive, self-appraisal, anxiety) and respond to when someone has an eating disorder?

Text links

Chapters 1, 11, 13, 19 and 25 in Elder R, Evans K, Nizette D 2013 Psychiatric and mental health nursing, 3rd edn. Elsevier, Sydney

Websites

Centre for Eating & Dieting Disorders: **www.cedd. org**

Centre for Excellence in Eating Disorders: **http:// ceed.org.au**

Maudsley Parents: **www.maudsleyparents.org**

The Butterfly Foundation: **www.thebutterfly foundation.org.au**

References

Berkman ND, Bulik CM, Brownley KA, Lohr KN, Sedway JA, Rooks A, Gartlehner G 2006 Management of eating disorders. Agency for Health Care Research & Quality, US Department of Health and Human Services. Available at: **www.ahrq.gov/ downloads/pub/evidence/pdf/eatingdisorders/ eatdis.pdf**

Bidwell Smith C 2012 The rules of inheritance. Hudson Street Press, New York

A final word

The St Leons bravely shared their family's agonising story of their young daughter, whom neither they nor the specialist mental health team could save.

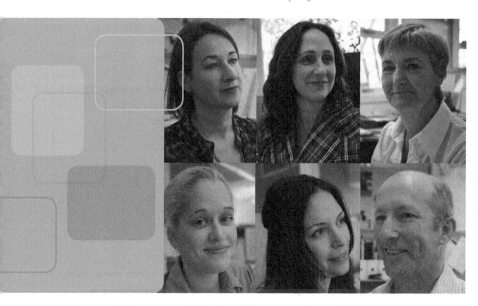

Collaborative practice

Introduction

The Eating Disorder Outreach Service (EDOS) is a multidisciplinary team that meets to discuss cases that have been referred to it from across Queensland. The EDOS team comprises:

- Elaine Painter, mental health nurse and team manager, EDOS
- Dr Warren Ward, Director, Eating Disorder Service and Chief Training Supervisor, Metro North Mental Health, Royal Brisbane and Women's Hospital (RBWH)
- Amanda Davis, state-wide specialist dietician, EDOS
- Carmel Fleming, state-wide specialist social worker and clinical educator, EDOS
- Rachael Bellair, senior clinical psychologist, Eating Disorders Inpatient Unit, RBWH
- Johanna Dalton, clinical nurse consultant, Eating Disorders Inpatient Unit, RBWH

View this story on evolve
http://evolve.elsevier.com/AU/
Nizette/stories/

Reflection

Listen to the team members' interaction to identify what data they are considering in order to develop a collaborative mental health plan.

Inquiry

Identify relevant issues impacting on Alice's psycho-social wellbeing. Make a table with three columns. In the first column identify the issues identified by the multidisciplinary team; and in the second column identify any issues that you think need to be considered as well. From the video and from your reading, in the third column identify strategies that may address needs.

Action

If you are interested in learning more about this complex mental health problem, the Centre for Eating and Dieting Disorders (CEDD) provides an e-learning course that you can access freely. The resource contains valuable information about:

- the roles of various health professionals
- assessment of people with eating disorders
- different therapeutic approaches
- management.

Websites

Academy for Eating Disorders: **www.aedweb.org/ Medical_Care_Standards.htm**

Australian & New Zealand Academy for Eating Disorders: **www.anzaed.org.au**

Beyond Blue Eating Disorders and Depression fact sheet: **www.cedd.org.au/uploads/file_292.pdf**

Mental Health Professionals Network: **www.mhpn. gov.au**

MH-Kids Eating Disorders Toolkit: **www.cedd.org. au/uploads/file_203.pdf**

NICE Guidelines UK: **www.nice.org.uk/guidance/ index.jsp?action=byID&r=true&o=10932#do cuments**

Text links

Chapter 23 in Elder R, Evans K, Nizette D 2013 Psychiatric and mental health nursing, 3rd edn. Elsevier, Sydney

References

McVey G, Pepler D, Davis R, Flett G, Abdolell M 2002 Risk and protective factors associated with disordered eating during early adolescence. The Journal of Early Adolescence 22(1):75–95

Prochaska J, Redding C, Evers K 1997 The transtheoretical model and stages of change. In Glanz K, Lewis FM, Rimer BK (eds) Health behavior and health education: theory, research, and practice, 2nd edn. Jossey-Bass, San Francisco

A final word

Elaine states:

I suppose if someone hasn't worked with a client who has an eating disorder before, there's a few things that are good to know. First, we tend to externalise the eating disorder from the patient, so we might say, 'You're really struggling with the eating disorder this week' or 'The eating disorder is making things really difficult'. Externalisation is a narrative therapy technique that is really helpful when talking to patients and their families. It separates the eating disorder from the person. It can sound a bit strange at first when you say, 'The eating disorder is giving you a hard time' or 'That's the eating disorder talking', but you do get used to it pretty quickly. There are also some simple things that can really upset our patients; for example, it's never good to say 'You're looking well' or 'You're looking better' or 'You're looking more healthy'. That can really put out a patient with an eating disorder because they feel like you're making a comment about them being bigger or fat, so it's better to say, 'How are you feeling today?' and comment more on the emotion rather than any kind of physical comment.

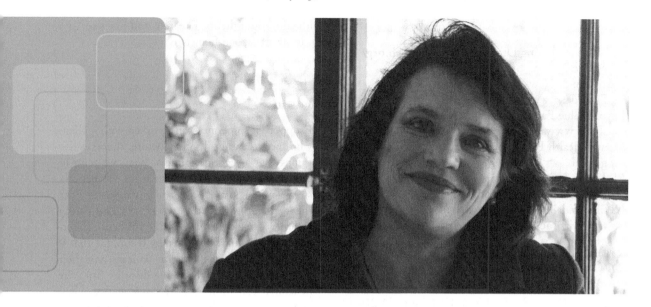

Kay's story: The social and physical impacts of alcohol

Introduction

Kay has endured more than 20 years of addiction to alcohol, from which she is currently 22 months sober. She has had an incredible journey that has included many physiological and psychological hurdles, but she is coming out the other side.

> View Kay's story on evolve
> http://evolve.elsevier.com/AU/
> Nizette/stories/

Videos

1. Kay's journey through alcohol abuse and recovery
2. Getting specific with interviewing

Reflection

1. Content-related questions: notice how Peta drills down on the problematic issues encountered by Kay. The objective for Peta was to produce a clear picture of the problem (whether this be alcohol misuse or disordered eating, for example).
2. Focusing on process: Peta demonstrates active listening skills that help Kay to speak openly about what could have been a very humiliating confession. Recall the elements of active listening. Make a note of how Peta did that.
3. Notice how Peta verbalises a non-judgemental stance while listening to Kay's experiences.
4. Notice how Peta perseveres in questioning Kay in order to elicit specific details about her alcohol consumption, triggers and antecedent behaviours.

Inquiry

While listening to Kay, use the social ecological model (see Figure 6) to identify and map factors that impact on (a) what maintained the alcohol abuse and (b) what supported her recovery from alcohol dependence.

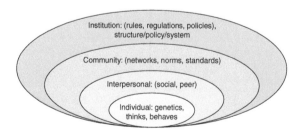

Figure 6 Social ecological model
Source: http://lsuagcenterode.files.wordpress.com/2011/07/social-ecological-framework.jpg

Action

Search the internet for a CAGE questionnaire and use this to assess Kay's alcohol consumption.

Websites

Alcoholics Anonymous: **www.aa.org.au**
Centre for Youth Substance Abuse Research: **www. uq.edu.au/health/cysar**
Hello Sunday Morning: **HSM.com.au**
Narcotics Anonymous: **www.na.org.au/ community/index.php**
National Drug and Alcohol Research Centre: **http://ndarc.med.unsw.edu.au**

Text links

Chapters 8, 20 and 25 in Elder R, Evans K, Nizette D 2013 Psychiatric and mental health nursing, 3rd edn. Elsevier, Sydney

Reference

Hayfield D, McLeod G, Hall P 1974 The CAGE questionnaire validation of a new alcoholism screening instrument. American Journal of Psychiatry 131:1121–1123

A final word

Kay is an amazing woman. Her honesty and bravery in sharing her journey into alcoholism are humbling. To have the courage and strength to pull herself out of a physical and psychological quagmire is inspiring. Everyone can change. We should never give up on people.

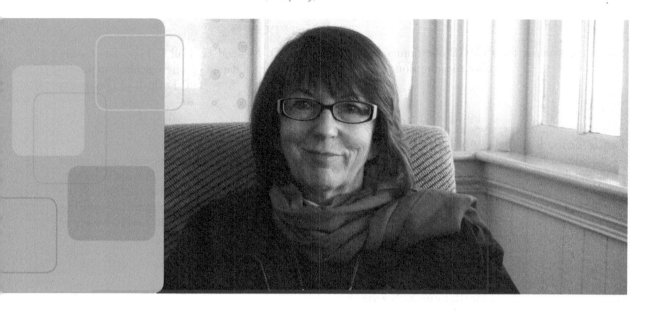

Colleen's story: Health education as core to mental health nursing

Introduction

Colleen is a mental health nurse and a general nurse. She believes that it is important to have both skill sets when working with people who experience addiction(s). She particularly uses her educational skills, because a large part of what she does is to provide education to clients and their families, both on an individual basis and together, about dependence, addiction and the physical, social and emotional impacts of substances on people. She also does a lot of group work within the context of her work environment, so sees the importance of having good group management skills.

View Colleen's story on evolve
http://evolve.elsevier.com/AU/
Nizette/stories/

Videos

1. Assessing alcohol intoxication
2. Adjusting the pace of treatment
3. Types of treatment
4. Loss

Reflection

As a student, if you are with a person who is expressing sadness and loss in this context, how can you show your compassion and bear witness to their pain?

Inquiry

1. What are the stages of alcohol withdrawal? Why is it important to intervene, even if the person is still showing signs of alcohol intoxication?
2. Identify some resources for psychoeducation around the safe use of substances, and substance abuse.
3. Using the Stages of Change Model (see Figure 7), explain why it is important to take things at the client's pace.
4. Why not implement aggressive treatment for alcohol cessation?
5. Research the use of evidence-based interventions relevant to supporting alcohol cessation, such as acceptance and commitment therapy.

Action

1. Look up strategies to assist people to express their grief, so that you can give people struggling with

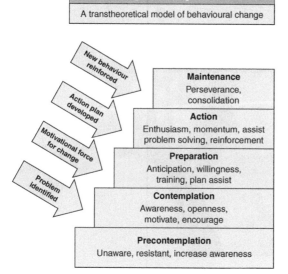

Figure 7 Prochaska and DiClemente's Stages of Change Model
Source: reproduced with permission of James Prochaska and Carlo DiClemente, www.prochange.com

grief and loss the tools to work with to express their grief.

2. Discuss strategies that Colleen suggests can be helpful in eliciting accurate estimations of alcohol use and surrounding stressors.

Websites

Acceptance and Commitment Therapy: **http://contextualpsychology.org/act**
Addiction Information: **www.addictioninfo.org**

AIHW: **www.aihw.gov.au/publication-detail/?id=6442467962**
Centre for Youth Substance Abuse Research: **www.uq.edu.au/health/cysar**
Mindfulness: **www.actmindfully.com.au/mindfulness**
National Institute on Drug Abuse: **www.drugabuse.gov**
The Happiness Trap: **www.thehappinesstrap.com/about_act**

Text links

Chapters 10, 20, 25 and 26 in Elder R, Evans K, Nizette D 2013 Psychiatric and mental health nursing, 3rd edn. Elsevier, Sydney

References

MILFA Substance use—Stages of Change Model. Available at **www.mifa.org.au/sites/www.mifa.org.au/files/documents/SubstanceUseStagesofChange.pdf**

Vercoe E, Abramowksi K 2004 The grief book: strategies for young people. Black Dog Books, Fitzroy

A final word

Colleen states:

> I think that in our society we have a view of what a person that overuses alcohol is like—there's a stereotype. Rarely does the person with the problem meet that picture.

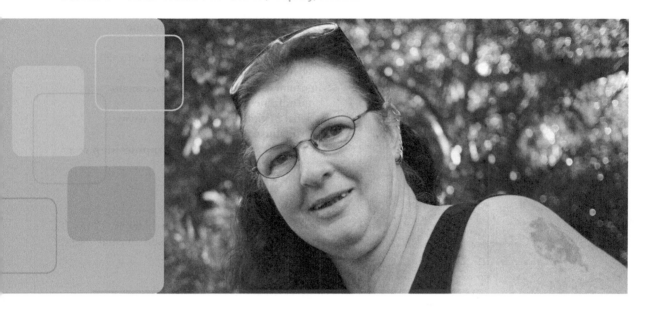

Zoe's story: Living with multiple selves

Introduction

Zoe is a woman in her 40s who has lived with the diagnosis of dissociative identity disorder (DID)—previously called multiple personality disorder—for 20 years. Throughout the interview you will hear Zoe talk about herself and her 'alter' personalities. To her, these personalities are different people and she does not know them well, although she has learned to communicate with them. Zoe does not know the cause of this disturbance to her sense of self, nor does she feel the need to find out the central cause. Zoe has managed to adjust and adapt to living peacefully and respectfully with the many different parts of her self.

Quick facts

DID is very different from dissociation generally. DID is a serious disorder. Dissociation is a common and healthy defence used in response to danger and is associated with memory loss and a sense of disconnection from yourself or your surroundings. Many people experience mild dissociative symptoms even when there is no stress or danger (e.g. daydreaming, not remembering a car journey or getting lost in a good book). When the defence mechanism is used involuntarily and with damaging, self-defeating outcomes, it is considered a disorder. Dissociation exists on a continuum with mild acts such as daydreaming at one end and more severe symptoms such as amnesia and identity alteration at the other.

View Zoe's story on evolve
http://evolve.elsevier.com/AU/
Nizette/stories/

Videos

1. Zoe's story
2. Triggers for switching
3. Cooperation is my goal

Reflection

1. DID remains a controversial diagnosis (Ross, 2003). Say, for a moment, that you believe that DID exists: what evidence supports the case? Now take the sceptical position: what evidence supports the case that DID is a fictitious disorder?
2. There will be many cases in psychiatry where the diagnosis is unclear or under debate. In fact, there are some who believe that there is no such thing as mental illness at all, that what matters is the promotion of peace, happiness and freedom.

Mental health nurses aspire to being empathic, non-judgemental and supportive, regardless of a person's diagnosis or readiness to engage in care. How would you describe the empathy that was triggered in you as you listened to Zoe? Why did you feel for her? What do you hope for her? How do you hope nurses will be when they are working with others who experience a deeply disturbed sense of self?

Inquiry

1. Alter personalities (or parts) are often brought into existence in order to serve some function for the person, usually following significant trauma (see Elder, Evans & Nizette, 2013, p 401).
2. What signs and symptoms of DID did Zoe speak about?
3. What are Zoe's strengths, and how might these benefit her whole adaptation and wellbeing?
4. What other functional 'parts' do you think might need to exist in Zoe's personality make-up for her to have survived and thrived in the world as she does today?
5. How is dissociation a coping mechanism? What is the problem with using dissociation?
6. Investigate what the terms 'switching' and 'triggering' mean. Why might a person with DID 'switch' to another personality? How might this put the person at risk of harm?
7. Why do you think many people with DID engage in self-harm? What function did self-harm offer to Zoe?
8. Thinking about common patterns of experiences leading to DID, what other life situations could be 'triggering' for people who have a diagnosis of DID?
9. Why do people with DID sometimes require acute care?
10. What factors facilitate recovery?
11. What, in the clinical context, might trigger people to dissociate?
12. How might nurses create an environment that is safer and less triggering for people?

Action

1. Go to the ISSTD online and find out what current therapies are considered world's best-practice treatment for DID.
2. Search online for the Dissociative Experiences Scale. Appraise this tool's benefits and limitations.
3. Research relevant care frameworks developed to assist nurses and the person to facilitate recovery (start with McAllister et al 2001).
4. Use the DID care framework to identify areas where the mental health nurse role could have assisted Zoe to adapt more promptly or successfully during her challenging experiences.

Websites

A reliable website providing consumer information: **www.dissociation-world.org.uk/dissociation**
Colin A Ross Institute: **www.rossinst.com/medical_papers.html**
International Society for the Study of Trauma and Dissociation: **www.isst-d.org**
Learn more about Zoe's experience at: **http://sarahkreece.blogspot.com.au/p/to-buy.html** and **www.abc.net.au/health/yourstories/stories/2010/06/17/2929421.htm**

Text links

Chapters 1, 21 and 24 in Elder R, Evans K, Nizette D 2013 Psychiatric and mental health nursing, 3rd edn. Elsevier, Sydney

References

McAllister M 2012 Positive skills, positive strategies: solution focused nursing. In De Chesnay M (ed) Caring for the vulnerable, 3rd edn. Jones & Bartlett, New York, pp 153–168

McAllister M, Higson D, McIntosh W, O'Leary S, Hargreaves L, Murrell L et al 2001 Dissociative identity disorder and the nurse–patient relationship in the acute care setting: an action research project. Australian New Zealand Journal of Mental Health Nursing 10:20–32

Ross C 2003 Dissociative identity disorder. Current Psychosis and Therapeutics Reports 4(3):112–116

A final word

Zoe has a final word of inspiration for future nurses:

> Even if you don't feel like you're an expert, the best strategy you can use when someone is in distress is to ask them what's going on.

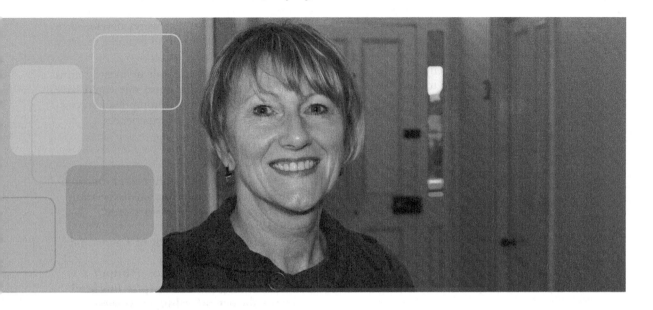

Jay's story: Being non-judgemental

Introduction

Jay is a mental health nurse who works in a service that supports victims of violence and crime and their families. The people who have offended have been diagnosed with a mental illness, and the service also works with their families.

View Jay's story on evolve
http://evolve.elsevier.com/AU/
Nizette/stories/

Videos

1. Mental illness and violence
2. It's about balance
3. Everyday people, extreme circumstances

Reflection

1. For nurses and health professionals working in the service, Jay says that it is about not taking sides—it is about being objective. Jay talks about the graphic stories she and others hear and the feelings of anger, guilt and grief of the victims and their families.

2. Can you think of ways that would assist you to maintain perspective and objectivity in this type of setting?
3. Victims of crime and violence live and work in our communities. What type of services could be helpful for them, and what kind of community do we need to keep people safe? (Consider the safety of both offenders and victims.)

Inquiry

1. Jay believes that the perception that people with mental illness are more likely to commit crime is disproportionate to reality. Compare/observe the level of violence or crime in the general population to the population of people with mental illness (review newspaper reports/news stories/research literature).
2. Explore the notion of unconditional positive regard. How does this relate to what Jay is saying about her role?

Action

1. Refer to the section on clinical supervision (CS) in Part 2 of this resource and discuss the role of CS in this setting.

2. In efforts to support victims Jay talks about a 'covert' assessment, as the victims are not patients but ordinary people to whom an extraordinary event has occurred.

3. What sorts of issues need to be monitored to ensure that victims and their families receive the necessary support?

Websites

Mental Health and Crime Information is available at the Australian Institute of Criminology: **www.aic.gov.au/crime_community/ communitycrime/mental%20health%20 and%20crime.aspx**
www.aic.gov.au/en/crime_community/ communitycrime/mental%20health%20 and%20crime/mental_health_cjs.aspx
UTAS Criminology Research Unit: **www.utas.edu. au/sociology/CRU/cru.html**

Text links

Chapters 1, 22 and 23 in Elder R, Evans K, Nizette D 2013 Psychiatric and mental health nursing, 3rd edn. Elsevier, Sydney

References

Gildberg F, Bradley S, Fristed P, Hounsgaard L 2012 Reconstructing normality: characteristics of staff interactions with forensic mental health in-patients. International Journal of Mental Health Nursing 21(2):103–113

A final word

Jay concludes:

> We don't engage and take sides. We try and balance the information so that we help the victim work through their trauma and provide an understanding of mental illness and the system.

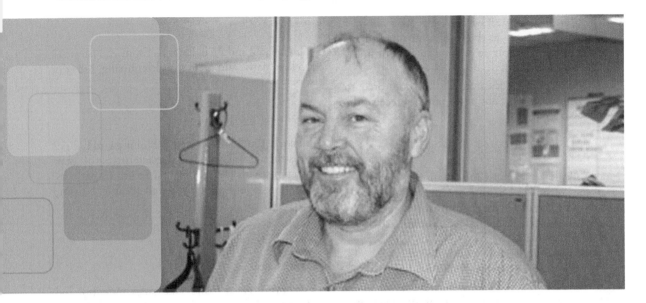

Bill's story: Cultivating a therapeutic milieu

Introduction

Bill Bailey is a mental health nurse who works as part of the crisis team on-site in the emergency department at Canberra Hospital, doing mental health assessments—ordered through the courts by a magistrate, directly from the police, through self-presentations, GP referrals or referrals from the emergency department. Bill has a Diploma of Forensic Psychiatry. Prior to his current position, he worked in the forensic unit at Long Bay Hospital, establishing a female high-dependency ward for the female clients dotted around New South Wales prison services with no access to forensic mental healthcare.

View Bill's story on evolve
http://evolve.elsevier.com/AU/
Nizette/stories/

Reflection

Bill tells a story of a nurse who demonstrates their availability to clients in a way that is appropriate for the setting. What are the messages from this description that could inform your future practice?

Inquiry

1. Developing a therapeutic milieu used to be a core mental health nursing skill that all mental health nurses learned about, but this seems to have slipped off the agenda recently. These days there seems to be greater concern for the provision of security over a therapeutic environment that cultivates personal and interpersonal safety. Bill hasn't let the concept of the therapeutic milieu slip off his agenda. How does Bill manipulate the environment to be therapeutic?

2. Look at other environments that you have worked in and suggest how you could make the environments supportive of therapeutic processes.

Action

1. As you listen to Bill talking, make a note of the unique aspects of his role. Use your list and map this to the 16 forensic psychiatric standards (see below).

2. Prison culture is a complex environment where there is tension between therapy and security. Read the brief paper on Tasmanian prison culture (see Resource 2 below) and make a mind-map of the dynamics.

3. It takes people to challenge dehumanising cultures. As Bill speaks about the daily life of prison culture,

he demonstrates examples of 'intelligent kindness'—the enactment of human contact, using examples and being inclusive are all ways of creating an environment that cultivates change. Do an internet search for the book *Intelligent kindness*. While much of this book provides examples of how the healthcare system can lack kindness, what lessons are conveyed both in the book and in Bill's insights for how systems can be humanised?

Resources

1. Forensic Mental Health Nursing Standards of Practice 2012

Forensic mental health nursing is a subspecialty of mental health nursing, rather than a subspecialty of forensic nursing where the focus is more victim oriented. The Forensic Mental Health Nursing Standards of Practice 2012 (Martin et al 2012) must be considered as building on the nursing standards, codes of practice and ethics that are common to all nurses, and further building on the Standards of Practice for Australian Mental Health Nurses 2010 (ACMHN, 2010). The Standards are outlined below; the full version is available from the Victorian Institute of Forensic Mental Health.

The forensic mental health nurse will:

Standard 1: Structure the treatment environment to integrate security with therapeutic goals.

Standard 2: Apply knowledge of the legal framework to service delivery and individual care.

Standard 3: Conduct forensic mental health nursing practice ethically.

Standard 4: Practice within an interdisciplinary team that may include criminal justice staff.

Standard 5: Establish, maintain and terminate therapeutic relationships with forensic service patients using the nursing process.

Standard 6: Integrate assessment and management of offence issues into nursing care processes.

Standard 7: Assess for the impact of trauma and engage in strategies to minimise the effects of trauma.

Standard 8: Assess and manage risk potential of forensic service patients.

Standard 9: Manage the containment and transition process of forensic service patients.

Standard 10: Promote optimal physical health of forensic service patients.

Standard 11: Minimise potential harm from substance use by forensic service patients.

Standard 12: Practise respectfully with families/carers of forensic service patients.

Standard 13: Advocate for the mental health needs of forensic service patients in a prison or police custodial setting.

Standard 14: Support and encourage optimal functioning of forensic service patients in long-term care.

Standard 15: Demonstrate professional integrity in response to challenging behaviours.

Standard 16: Engage in strategies that minimise the experience of stigma and discrimination for forensic service patients.

Source: Martin T, Ryan J, Bawden L, Summers M, Maguire T, Quinn C 2012 Forensic Mental Health Nursing Standards of Practice 2012. Victorian Institute of Forensic Mental Health (Forensicare). Available at **www.forensicare.vic.gov.au**

2. Prison culture and the pains of imprisonment

White R 2003 Prison culture and the pains of imprisonment. Briefing Paper 1. Criminology Research Unit, Hobart

Websites

Justice Health NSW: **www.justicehealth.nsw. gov.au**
UTAS Criminology Research Unit: **www.utas. edu.au/sociology-social-work/centres/ criminology-research-unit**
Victorian Institute of Forensic Mental Health: **www.forensicare.vic.gov.au**

Text links

Chapters 1, 5 and 22 in Elder R, Evans K, Nizette D 2013 Psychiatric and mental health nursing, 3rd edn. Elsevier, Sydney

References

Ballatt J, Campling P. Intelligent kindness: reforming the culture of healthcare. RCP, UK

Martin T, Ryan J, Bawden L, Summers M, Maguire T, Quinn C 2012 Forensic Mental Health Nursing Standards of Practice 2012. Victorian Institute of Forensic Mental Health (Forensicare). Available at **www.forensicare.vic.gov.au**

White R 2003 Prison culture and the pains of imprisonment. Briefing Paper 1. Criminology Research Unit, Hobart

A final word

Debra Nizette says:

> I really like how Bill makes mention of using a chair as a therapeutic device—a demonstration that the clinician is available, without being intrusive. This has particular meaning in the prison context where people feel that they are being intruded upon and observed all the time.

Debra suggests that all clinicians should be mindful of being seen to be available for consumers to generate the possibility of connection.

Transcripts

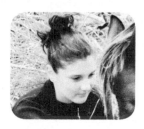

Makhala

Hi, my name's Makhala, I'm a Youth Brain Trust member with the Young and Well CRC. Basically what I want to help do is to improve the way young people with mental health issues are treated in the hospital system. I've struggled with anorexia for about six years of my life. I've been hospitalised for about two years out of that time. So when I was admitted into hospital on my first admission I was about 15 years old. I got hit with a lot of stigma, a lot of the nurses thought I was only doing it for attention and that, it sort of felt like they thought I was being childish by not eating and that it was easy to eat and the way that they put it made me feel like I was doing it purposely to hurt my family and my friends. Well this is definitely not the case for me, and not many nurses actually took the time to understand what actually caused my eating disorder, so a lot of people just judged me. Because I was admitted for so long it got to the point where people were just referring to me as a bed number. I was on special care on and off quite a lot. This was good and bad in some ways depending on who was looking after me as to how I was going recovery-wise. Some nurses would just sit there and they'd, I don't know, they'd give you this look that they didn't understand and they didn't want to understand. Because I was in a paediatric ward, I wasn't in a mental health facility, I was surrounded by sick kids as well and you sort of get put below all the other people because they just think that you are doing it to yourself you are not actually sick, you can make yourself better and that, yeah, they just don't understand.

You are made to feel like your problem isn't as big as everyone else's problem and these people have no idea what I went through and yet they feel like they had the right to judge me. It kind of gets very, I don't know, you don't feel like you are worth anything and when you are struggling with your own problems and you are made to feel worse in a place where you are meant to be getting better, it makes it pretty hard to recover.

And I guess after being in the hospital for the 10 months, you kind of, I don't know, I knew I could either live or die. It was at that moment where you have to choose. One of the nurses, I don't know if it's legal or illegal, but she took me out to see one of her friend's horses, because she knew that I liked them, but I wasn't really able to be around them. That was kind of the thing that changed for me was that, it's kind of hard to understand, but it was like when I was around the horses it was like I was actually happy for once. I could, yeah, I would feel like I was myself again and that's all I really needed because the whole time I was in hospital I was made to feel like I was a number.

It made me feel like I was a person again, and when I was with the horses, or when I was just having fun and being me, I wasn't so much focusing on the eating disorder, whereas when you are in hospital that's all you have to focus on.

I like helping other people. I help out a lot in the community. I'm actually planning on doing a horse-ride in August from Rockhampton to Brisbane to raise awareness for Rural and Remote mental health. Basically by me helping other people I feel like I have worth again …

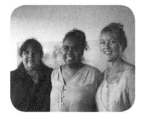

Jennifer, Anne and Christine

1. Working with Aboriginal people

Jennifer: My name's Jennifer McClay. I've been a mental health nurse for over 33 years. I've been here on the Sunshine Coast for the last 15 years and I've been working with the Aboriginal and Torres Strait Islander community for the last 10 years. I work on the Cultural Healing Program, which is Indigenous Mental Health, Queensland Health. We're a specialist service within the mainstream mental health. I work with my two health workers, Anne and Chris, and we work exclusively with the Aboriginal and Torres Strait Islander community and their families—if they're not indigenous we still work with them because it's a very holistic approach. We have an early intervention prevention model of our service, which is quite different to mainstream. It gives us the opportunity to get in very early and prevent issues. One of the criteria or the only criteria really to get into our service is to be at risk of a mental illness.

What we know of other services is often they have an Aboriginal health worker sitting in isolation and those traditionally haven't been very successful because they haven't had the support of a mental health service or other colleagues. There's a high turnover rate. With our service we very much value the Aboriginal health workers, they're a vital component to the program, you can't work with a community or a family without an Aboriginal health worker and so we sit together and we co-case manage. So we do everything together, so that we are culturally and clinically competent. Every time we visit somebody we go out; we don't do triage over the phone, that's really important. The community has direct access to us via our phones so to refer to us they just need to phone in or a GP phone in or family member and we will contact the person and negotiate to go out and see them.

Everybody knows the story and everybody can respond to whatever might be a situation the day and the other really important part is about tell your story one time, so it's not tell your story to me then tell your story to the health worker, then tell your story to the doctor or another clinician if you come back to the service. It's just tell your story once and we will then share that story, we'll write it on a document and we will share it with the doctor so that there's not that constant repetitive story telling and traumatising and things like that so that's a really successful part of the program.

It is a unique program. There have been other areas that have attempted to emulate what we do but just for lack support I guess for those programs to really be able to get up and running. There's no clear model of service at this stage for indigenous health service provision. We're hoping that we're able to contribute to that discussion quite a lot and there's been a lot of interest in our service and how we run. It has been a model service for the state in the past and often when we're talking to the Aboriginal community whether that be in health or community itself they really love the program and know that this is working really, really well so we're hopeful for the future I guess.

Christine: My name's Christine May. I'm an Aboriginal mental health worker with the cultural healing program. I'm a Wiradjuri woman from New South Wales.

I really enjoy my job, I love my job, I love my community whether it's your traditional community or the community you've grown up in or the community that you're now living in. It takes a long time to start establishing yourself in an Aboriginal community even if you're an Aboriginal person because they've got to suss you out, they've got to check you out and there can be lots of stumbling blocks in the beginning for us as Aboriginal people and working in mental health there's all that mistrust around mental health and all that stigma associated with it.

I love my job because I love to see my people healed, I love to see them go on, I'm very passionate about them going on and having a better and healthier life. I do have a degree in mental health and Aboriginal health and that's part of why I did that because to gain a better understanding around mental health because it freaked me out in the beginning so I needed to gain some skills and a better understanding and hopefully it's given me that.

I've seen a transformation even since when I started with the clinicians we work with have gained a better understanding, have better cultural practices when working with our people and have more compassion and understanding.

Anne: My name's Anne Humbet and I am an Aboriginal mental health worker and I work alongside Chris and Jennifer in the cultural healing program. My background is in aged care nursing and I've been a part of this community probably 15 years now and when I left aged care nursing I mainly left there because I wanted to work with my community.

Anne: Aboriginal know when you're fair dinkum, it's just about listening, it's about respect, it's just about being yourself really and people will know that, don't be scared of Aboriginal people, there's nothing to be scared about, it's just about acknowledging them and listening and acknowledging the culture.

Christine: Aboriginal people are loving people, kind people but we've also got an inbuilt fear and mistrust in us. Alleviate that and have fun with us and just enjoy being with an Aboriginal person, don't be scared at all and wherever possible engage with an Aboriginal health worker whether it's a mental health worker or a generalist or a child worker. If you have to see an Aboriginal person and there's no Aboriginal mental health worker around just ask if there is an Aboriginal health worker in that district, would they please be able to come out with you and you'll find they'll probably really enjoy going out and will respect you more for asking them.

2. Building trust and maintaining confidentiality

Jennifer: From a nursing perspective, cultural safety is about ensuring that the person's cultural heritage is acknowledged, that they are an Aboriginal Torres Strait Islander person and in the first instance you should try to have an Aboriginal person or Aboriginal health worker present when you're seeing someone of that cultural background. It's about acknowledging, it's about ensuring that they feel validated and safe, that really you're asking the health worker to vouch for you, to say this person's all right, it's all right to talk to this person.

   I always advocate that if you have an Aboriginal person there you should try and find, if there's a mental health indigenous health worker in the first instance; if there isn't there's usually a hospital liaison person who can come down and be with you, with that person's client's, permission, a family member, someone that may nominate. Someone so that they feel safe being able to discuss, particularly because we ask people very intricate parts of people's lives and we're expecting them to give over, particularly in the first interview and I think that's the other thing to remember is when you're working with Aboriginal people you may not get the story the first time or the second time or even the third time. Sometimes it just takes … you've got to build up that trust and rapport.

   You know, engaging with people, how you engage that's really important and learning how to do that is vital to be able to work with Aboriginal people, you know asking them about their family and where they come from and who's their mob and things like that is really important initial part of the process so that you can establish that relationship with the person.

   Confidentiality is a huge component of working with Aboriginal people and there are often concerns that when an Aboriginal person has another community member or a health worker that may be there, information will be spread amongst the community in other areas there has been an issue, so there has been that mistrust. What we do is we certainly upfront say, listen, we work for Queensland Health, our jobs depend on our confidentiality, so we very much explain about that right from the very beginning. Sometimes there are people who on the odd occasion would prefer a health worker not to be there and we respect that, so it's the person's choice.

   How we do our assessments is quite relaxed. It's a narrative approach really, it's just tell your story—certainly not sitting there with a document, ticking and flicking and filling it out. That just won't work. So getting the person to tell their story and a really good way to do that is to do a genograph because that way you're asking them about their family and so that's really important so you're asking who they are.

   So they start telling the story from birth, or even before that—you know, grandma, where grandma came from, where parents came from, who's Aboriginal, who's not Aboriginal and so then bringing the person through that story from the beginning from their childhood: where'd you go to school, what sort of kid were you, on to when did you start work and what year did you finish school, what did you do as a job, and bringing them all the way through the story in a very comfortable non-threatening way and in that you can get an assessment. You bring them to the point of what has brought you here today … ?

Christine: Patience pays off because sometimes when an Aboriginal person's asked a question they have to take that in, absorb it and they process it all so that they know how to answer the question. I've been involved with a lot of people being assessed in accident and emergency and I've seen questions fired at them; luckily I've known these people quite well and they've given answers back to doctors that totally wasn't related to why they're there and so the doctor's taken that and moved along with that and I've had to say, hang on a minute, like this is what he's really trying to say and the doctor said I'm not asking you and I went, well then you're not going to get a truthful answer.

   A lot of times our people will say yes when they mean no and because they don't want to be seen as not understanding what's been asked of them. Sometimes they will become really quiet after asked a question:

you have to allow time, they need to really process it and get it out the best way they can. So don't come in asking question after question, just relax and take your time so that they feel safe in what the answer they're going to give you, they don't feel silly or think you might think they're a bit silly.

A lot of the time we will try and call them back ASAP or our clinicians just to touch base and say, you know we'll get a health worker to give you a call because if you don't respond then tomorrow the crisis, the immediate crisis they're in which may not be related to their mental health but it might be around food or shortage of food for the children or something, that quick response is how you will start engaging because they think, they're interested, they care, so you've made a point first there.

We get a lot of people that will contact us with all their issues. It could be that they're going to become homeless or that they've moved into the area and they don't know anyone, they don't know, they need a bit of help with you know some food or getting the bond together or knowing the processes for this community so they will contact us. We don't turn anybody away; we're a mental health service but we do holistic mental health in line with our culture whether it's from my culture or from Anne's culture or it could be from Western Australia from the Nyungar people or you know Tasmania where the Palawa people and we will try and contact their communities with their permission just to get a bit of information about, not them in particular, but about their culture and the ways of working in their community so that we can gain some skills on better being able to engage with the people that come to us.

3. Listening to Aboriginal people's stories

Jennifer: There was one lady that we had, she was referred to us, the story was she was crying all the time, she wasn't sleeping, she was really sad, she was depressed, so we went around. I went around with the health worker and she was very sad and she was crying and she was depressed but the health worker that I was with at the time said, well could there be any other reason that this might be happening and she couldn't really identify and he got permission to ask the family and so she said yes and so we contacted a family member. Now this was over a couple of days so we didn't rush. She was hearing … when she was awake at night she described that she was hearing all these children calling out in the middle of the night and it was keeping her awake and she was tearful etc and when the health worker checked with her family, she had taken a child away without permission from the community and the family member said she has probably had puri puri put on her and that she needed to fix that.

Puri puri is like bad medicine, like most people Australian culture would know pointing the bone but there's all different versions of how that can be done and that is it can make somebody sick or make bad things happen to them or those sort of things … had I not had a health worker with me I very easily could have said yep, psychotic depression, probably needs an admission and medication—and that lady didn't need any medication.

Conversely I had another guy who was identified as unwell and we were doing the assessment and he started talking about cultural issues, like traditional things and why things were the way they were and who was against who. You know I, as a non-indigenous person and not in the know, I was intrigued by it, oh my goodness wasn't that interesting—and didn't think he had a mental illness at all. But my health worker went, hmmmm this fellow's talking like he's been through traditional law and he hasn't and he's got it all mixed up, yes there's some truth to that but he's got it mixed up: I think this man is unwell—and as it turned out he was very unwell and he needed to be hospitalised and treated and he recovered. So that's why it's really important because we can make assumptions either way and they can be wrong.

Go and attend some cultural events, be brave: NADOC's not just about Aboriginal people getting together, it's about community. Learn about the community that you live and work in; you know, that's got to be a start. You've got to find out who's around.

4. The need for cultural healing

Christine: We have a lot of people in their late 40s and mid-50s that are from the stolen generation which then you understand around the referendum in 67 and around like I was born and raised in New South Wales and where I was born and raised I was under the Flora and Fauna Act until I was 11 and so it did happen in our lifetime, so it does impact on Aboriginal people … wider Australia doesn't understand that it's still impacting on our lives today in many ways.

Anne: Chris is right, you know: that trauma is still there and I think for me, for my family, my mother was stolen generation: she was taken away when she was only really young and she was told by the person that she went to live with that her mother and her family didn't want her, she wasn't allowed to speak to them when she saw them growing up or anything like that and I took her back last year, she's 66 now, and I took her back last year and I found family and she still believed that until we actually heard the truth—that her mother did cry for every day, that her mother did miss her; and even when I think about that, that's upsetting for me and I tell my kids that story, that this is where mum came from, that she couldn't read and write and that she's really come along and made a life and she said to me one day, she said I've always been alone in life, I've always felt alone—so it does still tear me up when I think about it.

Christine: My grandmother's parents were taken to Blacks Camp in New South Wales in Wellington and later on placed on Nanima Reserve and because of abuse my grandmother was sent out to work at the age of 12 on one of the properties; because of the abuse being received [sic] by the property owner, physical abuse, sexual abuse, she ran away and she was in hiding for many, many years. We didn't know this!

Anne: It's about working together really, you know not doing it one person going this way and one person going that way or one person saying we should be doing this for those people; and I think it's about working together and striving for the same goals; and it's about Aboriginal people, it's about their health and it's about moving forward and I think we can only do that together.

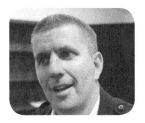

Toby

Working with people from ethnically diverse backgrounds is really a core part of working in South West Sydney: it's such a multicultural urban environment. I think it's a real melting pot in Australia as far as sort of the diversity of the place, and so it's very important to have some … some cultural sensitivity when it comes to working with people.

I have an interesting personal background which I bring to it, having relatives who are from different cultures, which I think probably helps me to feel a little bit more comfortable working cross-culturally, and I also just always keep in mind my own bias and my own sense of integrity I guess. I … I … one of the key things I try to do is not to become something I'm not. So working in an environment like this where I'm not sure if you can pick up the background music of the youth centre here, but it's very sort of loud and there's often dance here and there's often people from all sorts of different cultural backgrounds here that are quite young and funky, and I'm not young and funky, and so I … I don't try to be young and funky. I just try to kind of be myself and to maintain that perspective of a learner with the people as well. So, so when I'm … when I'm … when I'm working with patients, no matter where they come from, I'm always looking to learn from them. I often have patients say to me that one of the differences between seeing myself as a mental health nurse and, say, a psychologist they might've seen is the teaching aspect. They feel like I often teach them some stuff, which is kind of worthwhile. However, I could just as easily say to them, well you know wow and you teach me too you know—just about every patient does, so it's kind of one of those fun things; one of those rewards that you get from your mental health nursing is that you get a lot back.

How many people do I see who have a trauma history? Wow, that's a big question. Look, off the top of my head: you know when, upwards of … upwards of 60%, and if I'm working with the Aboriginal community it's upwards of 75%. It's a really … it's one of the really outstanding features of the Aboriginal community is that they have a very high level of trauma, interpersonal trauma and all sorts of other trauma that occurs that they just kind of take for granted, they're not even kind of aware of it, and you're sort of talking with the person and then they'll sort of refer to this time when their grandfather picked them up by the neck and threw them through a wall when they were little as if it was just kind of the norm, and that's one of the sad features, one of the challenging features of working with indigenous communities; and then, when you work with homeless communities, I mean there's been studies done in the inner city of Sydney which show that … I mean, there was one study done by Potter Teeson and Burick in 2001, and the reason I know that is because I sort of paid a lot of attention to their research. But I mean they had a study and they interviewed a cohort of like 500 homeless people, and of the women that they interviewed who are homeless it was a remarkable statistic that actually 100% of them had experienced trauma. Physical assault trauma you know. I mean I've … I don't think … the reason that stands out in my mind is because you read all these research articles and I've never read one that had 100% of anything. It was bizarre; it was quite extraordinary. So, you get a lot, you get a lot: when you're working with vulnerable populations you get more trauma.

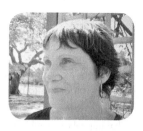

Bernie

My name's Bernie Waterhouse. I'm a person with a lived experience of mental illness. In 1991, at the peak of my career when I was personnel manager for a huge organisation, I became very unwell, psychotic. My family was really worried about me so I was taken to a private psychiatric hospital where I was diagnosed with schizophrenia. I spent the next five and a half years as a continuous inpatient in that hospital, without a day out and the only concern was my mental illness. The fact that I was a mother, a sister, had been a worker, just all went out the window.

I had no memory when I came out so it was like a child being dumped. You know, there was no community support and just the whole experience was very degrading. It was about power and control. I didn't have any input. There was no hope. I kept hearing that I had to come to the dreadful realisation that I'd always be unwell and always be in hospital, in and out of it, that my insight—I saw it as insight but they saw it as delusions of grandeur—that I could get well, I could study and I could get a job, were seen as delusions or grandiose ideas and I've done all those things but at that time it was just so degrading and so condescending, the care and now the reasons I moved to recovery or wellness. I find recovery a very confusing word for staff, consumers and families. It's like they've taken this word and given it a meaning that's just a different meaning for different people.

Like some people think, oh I've recovered, I can go off my medication, or I'm recovered, I should be working, and it's not that. It's about having a life where you can live with your symptoms and be a part of your community and it may be just a better quality of life or it may be complete wellness. I think when I look back the things about the staff, there was a lot of control and it was quite regimental—as I said, any insight I had was seen as rubbish, you really just had to do what you were told—and I think now I work in Queensland Health and the reasons I moved to wellness were being able to surround myself with people who gave me hope. They could see through all that darkness. They could see a little bit of light and even though I had been institutionalised and my expectations were that if there was anything wrong—it didn't even have to be anything to do with my mental illness—I'd be on the phone and I'd be ringing my case manager or my psychiatrist and saying, this is happening and my expectation is … I just put it out there and everyone else would fix it and I think the system did that. It made me dependent, it made me irresponsible and when I had people surrounding me who actually looked beyond the darkness, looked beyond the bloated body from medication and the sort of slur and all that.

When they could look beyond that and see I had some interests and I talked about maybe getting a job or maybe I could go and do this, the people that picked up on that and gave me choices that were meaningful, were the people that really aided my recovery and the people that listened. You talked about people listening, you often ask people, especially staff, to listen and they immediately go into why you shouldn't feel the way you feel or they go into what you need to do, like just go and lie on your bed for a while, where, as strange as that is, they haven't done what you asked; they haven't just listened. Yes, the end result might be you just need to go and lie on your bed, but if you can come to that decision and have some control—and I think now consumers, the carers and family having a say in their treatment, being involved, even when they're really, really unwell, being able to even talk about their symptoms, talk about the medication they're taking, involve them right from the start and give them some personal responsibility, like I want to know if you're feeling more unwell—this person will get well. And what are we doing?

What are we doing that makes that person not get well? Are we making them dependent? Are we not believing in them and their ability to move towards recovery, because if the clinicians and doctors don't believe you can recover, when you're really unwell, why would you believe it if they don't? It's just when you've got people saying oh you'll never be alright, you'll always be on medication, you'll always go in and out of hospital, it's hard to fight that. So I think now, I think I'm the luckiest person in the world because to be in the system for 12 years and get out of it takes a lot of effort.

I remember asking my sons, what was it like for you when I first became unwell? What was that like when you saw me in hospital losing my memory, sort of like a vegetable hardly able to find the bathroom? And my eldest son just said, 'that person in the bed wasn't our mum. That person was someone really unwell and we were just waiting for our mum to come back'… so I was just very lucky to have that support when I came out, yes.

Just always look for the little bit of light in that darkness and listen. Listen to what people are saying. Look at their verbal and non-verbal communication. Just believe in that person that if they have the proper support and the proper care that they can move past the crisis, because you're seeing them in crises. You're not seeing the person as they really are. Mental illness is only a part of that person and often only for a limited amount of time, when they are having that episode. So look for the light and believe in their ability to move towards wellness.

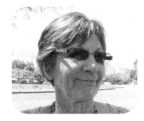

Jean

After quite a number of episodes over quite a number of years here in Queensland, Daniel had moved up here—he … on one hospitalisation, a different psychiatrist decided to try him on lithium, and that was a real turning point for us. I can remember after probably 10 days of treatment, noticing this—my son's back. There's a part of my son that's in there. It's like I'd lost him, I didn't know who he was for some time. And that wasn't the be-all and end-all, but it was the start of a recovery journey.

He still doesn't have a job. He has tried. Employment's difficult to get. He has difficulty concentrating, and lacks motivation.

Dan is quite dependent on me. More than I would like, and my big concern now is what happens when I die. But the system is changing. It has improved. Carers are involved more now. We really have worked hard.

When we come to the very serious mental illnesses, the results can be devastating if there's no early interventions. And if carers are left by the wayside, which then leaves consumers to flounder and fall through gaps. I think we've got beyond that, but there's a long way yet to go. We need to get some more social housing supported. Employers that will take on those that don't, perhaps aren't as productive, but still have a place in our society. So I'm hopeful for the future. Where 10 years ago I was really … I almost … I did become a consumer. I have had to take antidepressants myself and seek help along the way because it's been a long, hard road at times.

Stigma can come from all sides. It can come from within the system itself, within hospitals and certain psychiatrists and nurses, registrars—there can be this element of them-and-us. Or closing the door on carers, and I've often felt people look at me as if this is my fault. And sometimes even comments that might allay to that—he's a spoilt child, or you should have done this, you should have smacked his bottom—more of this this, type of thing.

But that can come from friends and family a bit, too. You should be doing this, don't do this, don't do—that type of thing. But I think as importantly as a stigma that we can feel from other people, I know many consumers and carers who … one of the hardest things for them is their own stigmatising, they can—it's my fault, or—it's hard to explain it really.

I think the word 'inclusive'. Try to be inclusive. Don't just see your patient; try to think of this person as a whole human being who has a family. Who may be homeless, who may have a home to go to, who has some friends. Or had.

Maybe that's where that person's got to, you don't know that, you don't know where they've come from. And I would ask that you don't make assumptions. A little bit of talking. I've been in many a visit to my son in hospital, and nurses do not—many nurses, I did not say all—many nurses do not do anything other than take charts around and check and tick boxes that somebody's here. I've sat for hours with my son and I've watched other patients and nurses coming in, and I think, well, they probably don't want to come over, or that Daniel's got his visitor. But they don't seem to want to sit down, and maybe just have a chat. Can be quite healing for someone to sit and listen or converse. Just try to find out a few things. It can't all be clinical stuff, it needs to be a bit more holistic and inclusive. I know behaviour around people with a mental illness is very, very hard to perhaps understand or even to tolerate sometimes, but …

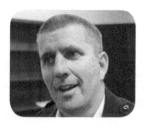

Toby

So when I reflect on my perspective of people who suffer serious mental illness like schizophrenia, you know bipolar disorder things, illnesses which have in textbooks written 10 years ago would've been described as chronically disabling illnesses that often people will need to remain on medication for ... for the rest of their lives. My perspective on their treatment and their likelihood of their likely recovery journey has really changed over the years. I think if you'd asked me 10 years ago I would've given you kind of a textbook answer: these people you know if they're diagnosed with schizophrenia, schizophrenal form disorder, schizo effective disorder and so forth, they're likely going to need medication for the rest of their lives. They're likely not going to be able to get a job, and they need supported housing, lots of support.

Now there ... there ... there is a lot of people who I see who, who I do think to myself their problems are so significantly insurmountable that when I look at it in the future, I guess they would fit that kind of picture. But more and more I have also been seeing a cohort of younger people who are able to access services like Headspace, like youth centres like this where they're able to actually get mental health treatment before the age of, say, 25, and I've seen them get better. I've actually ... I've actually had people who've seen two psychiatrists, they've seen me, they've seen psychologists, they've been put on medication and three years later they're off to university, off all their medication and there was no doubt that they suffered what the psychiatrist called schizophrenia, and their mother had schizophrenia and so forth, and they're at university studying, you know a full-time course without any medication.

So there is a cohort of people like that, so I think what we're seeing ... I think we're in a real, at the beginning of this 21st century we're ... we're at a transition point. I think the ... the ... the types of medication that we're able to give people, the types of therapeutic modalities that we're able to use with the people, and the service orientations that we're able to provide are really now making a difference that people back in the 80s, 90s weren't able to access, and so what they did was they went to the local pub, they went to the bar.

So I think with the increase in mental health literacy in the community generally too, we're seeing a real shift in the levels of hope that we can hold out for, particularly young people with these sorts of severe mental illness, so it's fun to be a part of.

Regarding what would I say to young mental health nursing students and what are they, what do they want to be thinking about, what do they want to be doing, I would say look, it's an exciting time to be part of mental health nursing, the sky's the limit. I mean, innovation is happening all around us and it's going to be fun to meet you.

Clinical supervision

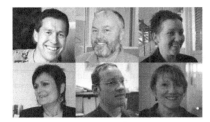

Christine: A clinical supervision is a professional development activity, where you set aside at least an hour to reflect on your practice and reflect on, in particular, your relationships with your clients. To ensure that you're working towards the well-being of the client, and that you're also conscious or more conscious of the processes that occur in therapeutic relationships. So the origins of countertransferential responses, so being able to recognise a countertransference in the therapeutic relationship and understanding where that comes from, how that happens, and being able to proceed more effectively in the relationship with the client.

I find clinical supervision's really important for me, and I always come away with a sense of having found myself much more in tune and in touch with my practice, and more thoughtful about working with certain people.

Todd: Clinical supervision is a particularly important part of especially psychiatric nursing practice. We're dealing with people with a whole range of emotional issues, or displays of emotion, and all of the interactions that you have carry some sort of emotional baggage with it. The way that you deal with or that you understand that emotional baggage is particularly important.

Through clinical supervision I can say for myself that I'm able to explore the interactions that I've had with people that I may want to revisit or may want to explore in an open environment that I can seek to understand or can put to rest the process of how I dealt with that person. I can critically reflect on how I dealt with that situation and either look at that in a positive light, or if I don't look at it in a positive light, look at the situation for how I may deal with it differently in the future, and how if I was to come across that situation again I might choose to act in that circumstance, rather than react to what's happened.

Mike: I just want to talk a little bit about the clinical supervision. Working with people with learning disabilities can be very frustrating.

It can become distressing and upsetting and we need an avenue to talk about that. Now your line manager isn't always the most helpful person in some circumstances when you're dealing with a difficult area of nursing, because they're also experiencing the same tensions and problems. Ideally, in clinical supervision you want to speak to somebody external to your service, possibly someone in a completely different profession, so you can work through some of the situations that you've experienced.

And clinical supervision is about personal development: it's about working through experiences that you've had; and it's also working through personal difficulties that you have in the role that you're carrying out.

Bill: But the culture of clinical supervision is often not seen for what I think clinical supervision should be about. They seek clinical supervision to address problems and 'this incident has happened at work and I need to go and talk about it at clinical supervision'. My belief about clinical supervision is about two steps before that: it is that you are constantly looking at areas of concern or at potential areas of conflict that you know they are there and it is about how you address them. I don't think you should go to clinical supervision solely after an event; you should go to stop events happening. I think the health officials have come a long way in resourcing and in getting clinical supervision up and running, but we still have to go a lot further and that is up to individuals to use it for what it is and not to use it as a debriefing after an incident.

Jay: Our service does hear some very disturbing stories from our victims. We also are privy to some quite graphic and descriptive material in regards to the offence and it's very important for us to maintain our objectivity and our investment or enrichment if you like quite separate. It's quite separate to become part of a story and to be enmeshed in that story and I think it's really important to understand clearly what your role is and what the expectation of your role is.

We're all human beings, so it's very hard sometimes to actually hear some of the things that we do and often we hear it not just once but again and again and again. So a very significant part of our work is to have supervision and we have very regular supervision to actually talk through some of those significantly disturbing stories that we hear. We have a very strong clinical supervision model and we have significant periods of time where we sit down and do our case reviews and we work through exactly what's happening with that person, what kind of service we're providing, how we're going to go about doing what we're going to do, what are the better approaches to interventions. We do have a multidisciplinary team and so we look at what are the best models and approaches to care that we can give to these people.

Toby: Alright, regarding clinical supervision nurse practitioner, where do you get clinical supervision? Well, because mental health is changing so much and … and when I did my nurse practitioner studies a few years ago I did a Masters through the University of Western Sydney, and none of the people taught me my Masters were nurse practitioners as far as I know. So there's a real dearth in sort of my ability to be able to access clinical supervision from a nurse practitioner. However, I do get very good clinical supervision from a couple of psychiatrists in two different clinics, and also I get it from a good friend of mine who's a … an academic professor of nursing at a university.

The types of clinical supervision that I tend to get with one of the psychiatrists, it's all about the clients, it's all about you know complex presentations, let's talk about the clients.

Rachel: So supervision is really, really important in child and youth mental health for any discipline. Nurses, I think it's only been in probably the last eight years or so, but nurses have really developed a strong clinical supervision background and I think it's made a really significant difference to the way we practice. It provides a lot of reflective practice; it provides capacity for somebody to talk about what the issues and challenges are that they're having with a particular person or with a particular therapy that they're doing and learn from that and build from that, and I guess at the end really be able to provide a better service for that person.

It also really helps individuals manage the feelings that they have that are brought up in working with young kids who come from really traumatised backgrounds and are facing sort of horrendous hardships and difficulties, and that's a really hard thing to go home with at the end of the day. So having supervision really helps put it all together and put it all into perspective and I guess at the end of the day realise that while what you're dealing with is really challenging, you're also doing a really wonderful job for these people.

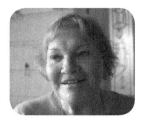

Claire

1. A day in the life

There was about 2000 patients, there was a male side and a female side, and mostly we worked … the female nurses worked in the female side of course and male nurses worked on the male side. There were two houses away from the main hospital, Orchard House and Forest House, and they were mixed, a very advanced idea in the early sixties.

We'd make sure they all got up, made their beds, took them down to breakfast and then the nurses served the meals. It would come in a big bain-marie and you served each patient. You knew what they could eat, what they were allowed to eat, what they liked to eat, and you just served the meal for them. And you tidied up and the bain-marie would be taken out and then you'd clean the ward. We have a big buffer so all the nurses—to polish the floors, all the nurses had quite slim waists. It was good exercise. And the patients would get in and help and then you might take them for a walk, take them to play cricket or tennis or something. We had an occupational therapy department and they could actually go there and work. They used to make Christmas crackers and sell them to the public. Some patients had other jobs. There was one lady called Martha and she would scrub the corridors. We had 20 miles of corridor altogether and they were wide enough for a car to drive through and still have room either side. And Martha would scrub about eight square feet a day but she knew everything that went on in that hospital and she got paid for it. Several of the other patients would go to work. Sometimes they could walk by themselves; sometimes you took them. They might work in the sewing room, in the kitchen, in the laundry and in the garden, depending on what they did. Some of them just sat in the ward and we'd try and encourage them to do some activity. A lot of craft work, we did a lot of craft work then.

I think the good thing the people were safe there. They didn't have many restrictions then. They were beautiful grounds. They could go and lay under a tree, they could go and do work and get money if they wanted to. And also we checked that they had food, their regular meals. They had to come into bed at a certain time, depending on summer or winter, it was earlier—summer time it was usually nine o'clock. But they came in and I think they felt safe with us. The worst things, we actually had padded cells there and as a first-year student you had to polish those padded cells. They were leather and you had to make sure the leather was all soft. The walls were a bit like a chesterfield sofa but the floor was like a dome, it was all very, very soft, horrible to be in though. There was only a little square for a window. I only every saw that used once.

2. The paradigm shift

The main changes that have occurred have been medications. There are so many good medications on the market without the terrible side effects that we've seen in the past. When chlorpromazine was introduced we noticed a big difference with the interactions with the patients. They opened up a lot more, they talked about things that we never knew about them and they were more amenable to doing activities with us. It just opened up their world for them.

The de-institutionalisation I thought would be good, but I think it was implemented a little quickly without being properly thought out. There didn't seem to be enough back-up in the community for some of the patients that were let out. A lot of them had lived in the institution for quite a long time and had had that constant support and some of them sadly they ended up back in because they hadn't had the support to live by themselves outside. Otherwise, I think it was a good thing. I think there are some patients that will always need to be in a hospital looked after that could never live by themselves, but they're very, very minimal. But I think it's very, very important to have that good support in the community. The patients they take their medication, they feel good, so they'll stop taking it. I don't need to take this any more, and then their behaviour gets out of control and the public are still very, very … sometimes quite unpleasant to people with a mental illness. They don't understand it. Some of them have no wish to understand it and they can be very harsh and it can create more problems. So the support in the community is very, very important.

Often the patients long ago didn't even know why they were there. I've got a mental illness. Now most of the patients are very well aware of what's entailed with their illness.

3. What I value about mental health nursing

I think if anybody wants to become a mental health nurse, go for it. It's the best profession I think because you're always thinking, you're always learning, there's no two people are the same, you've got their diagnosis but you've also got the person's personality, and it's always a challenge. You can see if somebody's medically sick but often you can't—well, you just can't see what's going on in the brain at times until you get to talk to that person or look at what their behaviour is.

You never stop learning no matter how old you are and it's just a very, very interesting profession and one that everybody I think should be proud of being in.

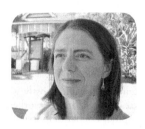

Lisa

1. My son's birth—a difficult time for me and others

I'm Lisa Bridle. I have three children: Amelia 19, Sean who's 16 and Declan who's nine, and Sean has Down syndrome.

We had a pretty intense experience when Sean was born, so he was at term but he'd stopped moving so I went into the hospital initially to be monitored and then because he was in severe fetal distress I had an emergency caesarian and when I woke up I guess all I could see was my husband's very grey face and he just said the baby has lots of problems. I guess before I could even take in the news the neonatologist came around and said your son's in ICU and there's no doubt that he has Down syndrome. All I can remember actually of that moment was calling out 'no!', so it was obviously a big shock and even though … I think I just felt very ambivalent about whether I wanted him to live or die at that moment. So he was very, very sick and what I remember then is being kind of wheeled past this baby covered in bubble wrap, ventilated, lots of wires coming off his body and then being taken to a shared ward where I guess the young mother who I was sharing that room with had lots of flowers and visitors and a healthy baby beside her bed. In those first few days I think I sensed a real sense of avoidance from some of the nursing staff, so they were very busy, they had something to do I think with my roommate but really the interaction with me was pretty minimal.

I think they felt very uncomfortable and I think the fact that probably the communication between the ICU and the ward wasn't good, so I think they didn't want to ask the wrong questions or almost even acknowledge that a baby had been born, so that was certainly my … so they kind of spent a lot of time on my caesarian wound and not very much time on any of the other kind of needs I had as a new mother. I guess, in contrast, the nurses in the neonatal intensive care unit I found fantastic and probably it was the kindness of some of those nurses that made a big difference in those first few weeks. Yes, I think what I remember of visiting Sean in the ICU is that it was a very intense and difficult time, particularly because I couldn't hold him. So probably about day three or four a very kind nurse said I really think you need to hold your baby today, and it was quite a rigmarole getting him out of the crib that he was in and getting all the tubes and things reattached, but it was a moment where I actually felt an intense sense of calm holding him, that everything from then on would be okay. So it made a very, very big difference.

Q. You say the nurses were very good at fixing up your wound and going about their business, but what did you need from a mental health perspective and what would have been enough?

Look, I think that's a really tricky situation because I think that lots of families' needs are actually different, so I needed a lot. I was someone who really wanted a lot of information, I wanted to read everything in sight and I think when I've spoken to other parents some people just really do want to be left in that bubble of not dealing with the diagnosis or dealing with too far down the future. It certainly did help … there are a number of nursing staff who'd had personal experiences and I found that helpful that they shared those, but I'm not sure that every family would feel the same. I think I just needed probably not to feel that my reactions were being judged, so there was a sense in which I felt that you couldn't be seen to cope too well, to be in denial, and also you couldn't be seen to be a complete mess. So I was aware of actually managing my own reactions, not for what worked for me but really kind of trying to avoid some sort of judgement and note taking and I did … I was actually one of these mothers that read the chart and there had been some, yes, some comments—parents seemed to be well or something—and I thought I'm not sure that I'm comfortable with having those reactions at a very intense and difficult time recorded.

2. A story of personal and family coping

I was very concerned about particularly how my family were coping and I felt like I had to manage their reactions by being very positive. I think I was anxious about what friends thought. I did feel, I guess, a sense of shame initially; it felt like my body hadn't produced the correct baby, and so I was dealing with that sort of sense of, almost embarrassment, that I hadn't produced the required healthy child, and, yes I think I just remember feeling probably distant from people and when I got home from hospital I was very isolated because Sean was on tube feeds, he was on oxygen, I was expressing breast milk up to probably eight times a day, so I didn't really get to go out very much and I think people weren't sure whether I wanted visitors, or I didn't want visitors or how to do that in a way that wasn't going to be an additional stress. So that was … it was an isolating time and I think I was very much preoccupied at that time by Sean having Down syndrome and all of his medical needs. So it was a difficult time for me to be in any way interested in maintaining those social contacts.

I was going to say I think looking back as well, obviously, that has an impact on your relationship, so I remember probably feeling that I was the person who was going to all the medical appointments, that my husband wasn't getting the latest round of bad news, and so I felt like he didn't really understand, and I think definitely we had the issues of each of us dealing with things in different ways. I felt incredibly guilty about not being emotionally available for my daughter and desperate because Sean was such a bad feeder, about his lack of weight gain. I guess probably having Amelia, having an older child was in many ways a saving grace because it did mean that I had to maintain some semblance of ordinary life for her. Like I needed to take her to child care, I needed to take her to swimming lessons or whatever we were doing at the time and as well for her, she didn't have the same preoccupation with Sean's diagnosis. I mean, I know that she didn't think it was completely normal to have big oxygen canisters in the bedroom, but it didn't have the same kind of emotional force for her, so it was a levelling and a balancing thing and over time I guess what I've seen is that she has just kind of grown up, as Declan has, with disability as part of our family story and it hasn't been a really negative thing at all; it's just been kind of ordinary. In fact, Milly would say that we were the most popular family at school because Sean was very sociable and outgoing and everyone knew him. He was also an embarrassing small brother so I think one day she wasn't so keen on him when he came: she went to school and he pulled out a very large pair of my underpants and put them over his shorts at lunch time and did a bit of a dance, so he also embarrassed the hell out of her. But generally I think it's been, I really think it's been a positive and enriching thing for siblings.

Mike

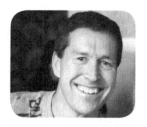

My name's Mike Musker. I'm a psychiatric nurse. I've worked with people with learning disability for many years. I was a charge nurse on a ward for patients with learning disability. Now we use the term 'learning disability' but the term changes over time and if we go right back in history, many patients are referred to as with perjorative terms like 'idiots', 'imbeciles' and 'cretins' and in those days that was an actual diagnosis. And today we have a system of labelling people which we call the DSM-IV and in that it talks about mental retardation for learning disability. There isn't always a specific facility for people with learning disabilities and they tend to come into the mental health services when there are no services available in the community or their behaviour has become particularly problematic for their family or their community. And an example of that might be a patient throwing stones at cars in the community, sitting down in the middle of the road, assaulting people …

Working with learning disability patients is a very rewarding experience. Many of them really enjoy the relationship they have with their nurse or their carer and they're very affectionate people usually and they really struggle to form relationships in the community. So when they meet a nurse and actually form a relationship, they really hold on to that relationship and value it very much, and you can reciprocate those feelings that the patient gives towards you, and that can be quite an enjoyable relationship. It's also a very challenging area of nursing in that you have to take on some difficult behaviours and help the patient manage those behaviours and particularly aggression. My experience is by treating the patient with respect and working through those behaviours with them again can be rewarding both for the patient and for the nurse.

Often patients with learning disabilities can be a harm to other people; they can be threatening, they can be hostile and aggressive. But they can also be self-harming, where they can pick themselves, bite themselves and also perform acts of self-harm.

There's also washing and dressing. Again, patients with disabilities they may neglect themselves, they may not wash. So they may need assistance with a routine in order to help them achieve that. There's sleeping. They often have difficulties with sleeping and poor patterns of sleep, which then reflects on their behaviour the next day, and their mood. There's eating and drinking. Many patients that I've worked with are obese: they have no control over their eating habits. They take medication which causes them to eat more, or some patients may not eat the same as you and I. They might gag on their food while they're eating, then they'd be off-putting to other people, so they may not be able to eat in social arenas. So they're some of the behaviours that we have to assist them to manage.

Eliminating is another issue. Many patients when they become constipated it can affect their behaviour, so again you have to make sure that the patient is basically … their health is holistic and that we're looking at every aspect of their care. Mobilisation—some patients are overactive and some patients may not do anything at all and you have to find a happy balance there. Working and playing, everybody needs to be occupied and have a bit of fun in their lives.

Communicating is a key aspect for people with learning disabilities and most patients will have some sort of social skills deficit, and that requires a whole training program around that.

Expressing sexuality is something that we don't always think about when we think of nursing. Often people with a learning disability won't have a sexual partner and they won't have formed relationships with the opposite sex. So that's something that you have to help them work through and sometimes discuss that explicitly.

When a person who is an adult behaves in a childlike way there can be a tendency to talk down to them as children and we need to avoid that because it only promotes that childlike behaviour. We need to be direct with our communication, we need to be clear and we need to talk adult to adult. And that brings the person back to the adult mode as well.

We had a patient who had a severe form of epilepsy and he would have serious epileptic seizures and that would involve him suddenly crashing to the floor and having a grand mal seizure. That patient used to build up to the seizure with the behaviours deteriorating over time. They would become more and more aggressive the closer they got to the seizure, and this would be over a period of around a month. The patient would be abusive, he would spit at people and he may also assault people, and he was very difficult to work with as an individual. However, we were able to put strict limits around his behaviour, which meant in the end he would actually display some of those behaviours less, and we worked with him over time to assist him in behaving appropriately with other people. Now that is a difficult case but again it can be rewarding if you can see the benefits that the patient is getting over time. Many of these patients are difficult to work with and the nurse will find it difficult emotionally interacting with some people. But again, there is reward in assisting that patient to live with other people.

If you write down what you value in life and we put those onto cards, and then we ask people to reflect on that experience and say, well, do our patients actually have a right to access those things that you like, like going to the cinema for example, like watching the TV programs, like going to bed when they want to go to bed, because in institutional care there's often an impinging on people's rights to the point where we're actually controlling their behaviour too much. So we need to be very careful what behaviours we limit and how we limit them.

With people with learning disabilities it can be quite a pessimistic outlook because their condition is lifelong, but that doesn't mean that you can't find the true potential of that individual. And you've got to be creative and look at ways that you can bring that potential and it's your job to work within a multidisciplinary team to promote that positivity.

When you work within a team, they can lack energy, they can lack ideas and you might have to motivate those people to start thinking differently to the way they currently do.

As a nurse, when you're working with people with learning disabilities, it's not always about work, about changing the patient's behaviour. It's also about providing some joy in the person's life, about entertainment, about occupation. So we would do things like games with the patients, like even playing Bingo, they were playing computer games, having a disco, playing sports. So it's not always about specific interventions on behaviour. It's also about having fun and some of the community trips can also be fun as well.

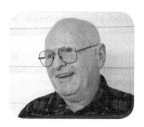

Gordon

1. Relating with carers

I just put all my faith in the doctors and in the children's hospital. These were not doctors that were mental health specialists; they were just general registrars that would assign her a bed in a hospital for her to be assessed by mental health staff within the hospital. From there we then started to get some feedback, but all that interfacing was with the mother. I was getting very little feedback until they wanted to interview the family one at a time because we had two other children.

A lot of the interviews with us as parents was with the mother during working hours, and occasionally they would ask for both of us to attend late sessions in the afternoon that fitted in with work because we were still trying to keep normal routine at home with two other children that were younger than Pamela was, so from that over a period of about six/nine months she was in and out of hospital, wasn't attending any sort of schooling for about 15 months in this time.

I saw a lot of mothers but I would hardly ever see any fathers. Now that is a big concern for me because there must be quite a lot of children out there where the fathers just do not get involved and I know from being on Minders, speaking to the mothers, most fathers haven't been involved and I find that shocking. Why? You've got to ask the question why doesn't a father get involved with their children's mental health issues. Is it because the father doesn't want to be involved or he feels as though there's a stigma, that he may be the cause of the problem and society today points the finger at the father too often.

They will interview the father maybe once or twice and then everything is then moved on to the mother as the prime carer, the emotional carer, because they look at mental health as an emotional-type health issue. They don't look at fathers as being able to give that. But children would look at a father as being stability, somebody to lean on, somebody to talk to when the mother becomes overemotional and depressed, and I think we lose that part of the healing process because we don't bring the father into it.

2. Family coping and caring

I found that I could openly talk about everything, whereas the mother, because of her previous experiences with her aunty taking her own life, found talking about emotions and mental health issues as a Victorian era: you kept it in the cupboard like a lot of families do. But I was quite open about it because of my previous experience when my own mother had depression and mental breakdown when I was a teenager and I was involved with that. So I had experienced the same situation but I found that I was coping with it a lot better than my daughter's mother was coping because she couldn't cope with that and she had the guilts: she found it difficult to talk about. And when one party is being so emotional and the other party is trying to be rational and be stability within a family, because you've still got two children that have to be looked after because they're younger in our family situation than the one that's going through the mental health, and we found that with our own children, they thought they could catch this disease, but it's not a disease, it's just an issue of the mind.

3. Gobbledygook

I think when it's a child and the parent's leaving their child behind at some health institution or therapy unit or something, where you're leaving them overnight or for weeks, the carers need to be given some very clear simple English basic understanding what their child has, without getting down to the medical terms. Just simple, 'Okay, your child has a mental health issue, we're not certain where it's at, what needs to be done yet but we will keep you informed. They're required to take this medication to get them to feel more comfortable with themselves'. That needs to be in simple terminology.

What I've found is that they use acronyms, medical terms which is for a parent that's in a state of stress that's all gobbledygook. We don't do it in simple language. If we give them a brochure you try to read it, it's all in medical jargon. The terminology is not simple English. When they give you ideas of how we're going to treat the child, some of the ways that they present it sounds as though they're going to abuse the child instead of comfort the child, because when you think about your own child, you don't want to leave it somewhere where they might get locked up in a room, the doors locked, they can't come out, it's like a prison. So the parent's going to think this is abuse.

Information wasn't forthcoming, that was a real big issue to me. There was no communications. Unless you asked the right question, you would never get the answers and because as a parent you're not in a state of mind where you can clearly think and you have all these different thoughts going through your mind ...

The key messages would be to listen to the carers, respond in simple English not medical terms, make certain that the person that you're talking to has picked up the message that what you're trying to explain, what the medical staff are going to be doing with the person that you're caring for, to listen to both parties of a family, which is the mother and the father, and also consider what effect this will have on the siblings of the person, because sometimes those siblings may be helpful in assisting the person that's suffering.

4. A father's reflection

I can relate to the young children of today because I see the youth today is our future tomorrow and if we can help them in their earlier life to get through mental health issues, they'll be a better person in the future and I can see that in my own daughter. She's an inspiration of where she's at today, but I know she went through a lot of pain in her teenage years. She lost her teenage years. She lost out on a lot but when I talk to her and listen to her talking about her friends of her own age, she's a much more mature young lady, has experienced life and can put up with a lot more pressure and stress than her own friends.

As a parent, as a carer, you've just got to be there to be that rock, that pillar to lean on and you don't have to put a lot of emphasis in talking to them. As long as you're there physically, I do believe a lot of children with mental health feel there's somebody to lean on, there's your comfort zone and that will allow the stress to ease out, but you don't have to talk. If they're in the home and you're there doing your own normal things and carry on as normal and they know that you're near, I believe that is part of the caring process.

I have a motto in my life, be consistent, persistent and do not discriminate. Now I use that through work because of the job I do as a contracts officer. I try to be persistent, I try to be consistent with how I deal with internal staff and external because I'm dealing with contractors and I treat everybody the same. I don't look at the internal staff as being better than the contractors and vice versa. I do believe the same thing should be treated when you're handling mental health issues. If you show some sort of stability in being consistent, persistent and not discriminating whether you've got a mental health issue or not, people will see you as a better person to maybe talk to, lean on.

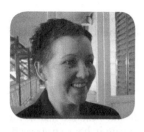

Rachel

1. Assessment issues in child and youth mental health

We receive the referral and that's either from the GP or from the school, sometimes it's the young person themselves or the family and we take all the information around what the mental health issues are for that person at that time and do a lot of collateral collecting as well. So we'll talk to the school or talk to the GP or talk to the school guidance officer, the school health nurse, people who have a lot to do with that young person and try to get different perspectives on what's going on for that person and ascertain really whether what's going on for them requires our service or whether we can look at another service that might be more appropriate to meeting their needs.

The priority would be a risk assessment, so we would really be looking strongly at whether that person's safe at that point in time. So looking at protective factors for them: do they have a lot of family support, do they have the capacity to call on family and friends or other services for support if they need it. Looking at access to means do they have family members that are able to help keep them safe and act appropriately and take them to hospital or take them to the GP if they're in a crisis or if things sort of turn really sour for them in that point in time. So we look at that really as the main assessment when someone's got risks or a considerable amount of risks. Otherwise, other assessments are looking at how they function: have they declined in functioning at school, are they still engaging in friendships and relationships, are they still getting up in the morning and doing what they would normally do; and looking at significant changes and if that's impacting on their current state of mind and trying to work out from there just their level of functioning.

Family is another really big area, so when you've got lots of family conflict going on at home, you've got parents who are separating, you've got parents who are unavailable or you've got other situations where there might be another child that's for whatever reason needing more attention or needing more input at that time and somebody feels left out, that can really have a significant impact on somebody's mood as well. Other sorts of stresses that I guess play a big part is to do with school, so the stresses involved in education and meeting the needs, especially kids in Year 12 with the exams and OP scores, and all those types of things really have a huge impact on somebody's ability to cope and ability to function.

General self-esteem is a big issue: a lot of kids don't have great self-esteem and don't have the resources to work on building that, don't have the resilience factors that other kids might have, so that can really negatively impact on somebody's general wellbeing.

When you're met with something traumatic or some hardship, if someone's had a really rough period of time, are they able to bounce back, are they able to build on that and learn from that in a positive way and gain strength to sort of move on and be a better person for it, or are they severely affected by it and can't seem to build on from it, can't seem to generate the skills that they need to realise that this is learning and then build on from that.

We do a lot of education, we do a lot of teaching young people themselves about what resilience is and how to build resilience. We teach them a lot about self-esteem and how to improve on self-esteem. We're able to really look at that particular person and pick out factors that we can see that their self-esteem is really good in some areas, maybe not in other areas, and build on the positives and focus on the positives but also really build on where their deficits are as well.

2. Young people and identity

Sexuality is a big area in child and youth mental health and an area that we're really just beginning to explore better than we have in the past, realising that there are such a diverse range of young people that present to our service and I guess in the past we possibly didn't ask those questions as well as we should have; so it's an area that has an obvious big impact on a young person's life, on how they deal with things and how they cope with things, because they've got dealing with their sexuality on top of that as well. So being really sensitive to the needs of a young person and providing appropriate support and I guess also realising that we're not experts in that field so having a really good knowledge of alternative services that are youth-friendly and able to provide the support that they need, that we can either refer along to or work in conjunction with to help that young person meet their needs.

There was a young boy who was 17 who had been referred to our service not that long ago. The GP had referred him for anxiety and it was only after really spending a lot of time talking to him about what are some of the situations that make him anxious and what makes him feel like he has concerns around anxiety that he was able to identify that he was gay and had really struggled with that his whole life, had just decided to come out and talk to his family about that, which wasn't well accepted. Some of his friends were quite supportive and quite responsive to it but he felt like he really needed some additional support in that area and building on some skills that he could help take with him in his life. Trying to help him build his resilience, trying to help him build his confidence around who he was as a person because this is him and he was proud of who he was. So trying to build on that, trying to make him stronger in that sense. We also referred him onto another service which further enhanced that and made him realise that he wasn't alone in this journey.

When you think of what youth-friendly is, it's a really broad topic as well because it can mean a whole number of things. I guess for our service we try to make it approachable, we try to make people feel like they're welcome, we're non-judgemental. We're warm and inviting people.

3. Consent and confidentiality

There are lots of challenges working in child and youth mental health which I guess is what makes it exciting to work in, but I guess some of the challenges are working with young people that have come from really compromised backgrounds and trying to work with that and trying to help them in a really positive way when sometimes there isn't a lot of positives to that person's life can make it really difficult, make it really challenging for you.

The legal aspects is quite difficult as well. There's a lot of issues around confidentiality so we have a really strong confidentiality clause in our service where we're very strong on our confidentiality. We let people know upfront, both the young people and the families, that what they say to us is confidential unless they tell us something where they're going to bring harm to themselves or somebody else and then we have to share that risk. The young people take that on board pretty well; the families take that on board pretty well as well, but it does come with its challenges and it does come with its do we tell somebody now or do we sit with this? And I guess that's a safety issue for the young people, it's a safety issue for the families and it's for us as well. So it can be tricky, you build up a really good trusting relationship with somebody and then they tell you something and you do sometimes feel torn as to whether you need to pass that information on. So it can be tricky from a personal perspective at times.

I guess the age of consent is also a really tricky one in child and youth mental health. Most of them aren't 18 yet, so what is that age cut-off where they are deemed a competent person to make their own decisions and to receive healthcare or to receive care when they may not have the consent of the family or if they don't want a family member involved. So we take all that into consideration. We often get a lot of kids who say that they don't want families involved, they don't want their parents to know about the referral and, depending on the situation, again depending on the risk factors and what's going on for them, we'll do our best to meet those needs.

Ultimately, at the end of the day, we're here for the young person and we want the young person's mental health to improve, to improve their functioning, to improve their performance, just to improve their health outcomes. So if by telling a parent is going to make things worse, then we would seriously consider whether that was the right thing to do or not.

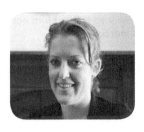

Nadine

1. Our family and dementia

I think mum's initial diagnosis was three or four years ago; however, looking back, I think it started maybe eight years ago. It certainly wasn't an area that I ever thought would impact upon my life. You don't really hear about dementia or Alzheimer's affecting anyone other than grandparents or people in their 80s, who suffer with some form of memory loss or mild memory loss as a part of ageing, going through your years, and I guess it's just not something that people generally worry about, because it affects the elderly at that later part of life.

Looking back, with my mum, and she initially … she went through loss of self-esteem, diagnosed with depression. She'd never had a history of any depression prior to that, never been sick, always extremely healthy, never overweight or ate bad foods or anything like that, so there was nothing to suggest that there is any factors that would contribute to such a horrendous disease. And then just the memory loss, and not understanding why that was occurring. I think initially it kind of went down to, she's just being silly, for some reason she's going through this period of time where she doesn't want to go out with her friends or she doesn't want to cook food, and mum would make excuses for that. She didn't want to cook because she's done it for the last 20 or 30 years, and now she thinks it's dad's turn. So we all thought that was pretty funny, go mum. Same with driving, she just decided she wanted to be chauffeured around, so again we thought, well if that's what she wants then that's fine. But looking back on it, that wasn't the case at all. Mum just didn't have that confidence in herself. And she was humiliated and, I assume, scared that these changes were occurring and instead of getting help and being open with that, and maybe proactive, unfortunately she wasn't and a lot of things went, not unnoticed, but it wasn't a major concern. And it should have been.

It's really hard to remember what was happening then, and the way I kind of look at it is I go, I remember my dad had leukaemia and I remember the day, the place, the time, everything, exactly how I felt, what I thought, everything, when he got that diagnosis, because it's such a common disease, but you also know that that can be fatal, the chemo, the treatment, the hair loss, that's sort of in society, so you know about it. And I think with dementia, because I knew nothing about it, it's really hard to try and remember, and it's not because I cared less; it was so sort of surreal and they just put such a positive kind of spin on it that you just kind of went, well, ok, we're not going to really see that much more change, it's going to be managing the behaviours we've got now. And she was still coping reasonably well, with some hints and just some minor assistance, that I just thought, well, ok, we're going to stay like this and she'll start to forget things, but we're going to be able to prompt that and to show her things, and so it really, at the time, it didn't seem that it was going to be anything major, like a fatal disease, or that she was going to die or anything like that.

In terms of our family journey throughout the whole process, it's horrendous. It's been horrendous. And obviously we'd get frustrated and we'd get angry, which is horrible to think back on and look at how angry, sometimes, we got. Because it wasn't her fault, but because we didn't understand how to deal with someone with dementia, or this memory loss she was supposed to be going through, we didn't really know what to do. And friends start to drop off. Her best friends stayed around, but even that got difficult, because she would accuse them of taking things or using her clothes or make-up or whatever it was. It was just extremely difficult.

And then the aggression started, which was like another phase. There are sort of phases that she worked through. So initially it was the crying, the not understanding what to do, and then it was the hoarding of possessions, not really being able to go out anywhere, not liking being in the car, trying to get out of the car, and the aggression was probably the worst part of it. Because you wouldn't know what she was thinking or what she thought you'd done to get a belt 'round the back of the head, or get something thrown at you. And it just wasn't her. She was never an aggressive person, but it was hard to try and deal with that behaviour. And then in England she got so aggressive at one point that they were concerned for family safety as well as her own, so she was admitted under the Mental Health Act and put in a hospital, and she stabilised. It was just a slight change in medication at that point, she was on anti-psychotics; they'd put her on risperidone, it was just kind of trying to manage the dose of that.

So she came out of hospital then, came back home; things seemed to be settled quite well, and then I came back to Australia. I was back for maybe three or four weeks, and then she got admitted again because of violence and aggression. She'd belted a couple of nurses. When I'd gone in, when I spoke to the nurses—I flew back to England, went to see the nurses to see what was going on, and they said that she wouldn't sit down. And I said, well, mum walks a lot. She doesn't like to stay still. And because they'd try to make her sit down, she had given them a quick slap across one cheek and then a backhander across the other one, so it certainly wasn't nice for the staff, but I think again it was that understanding that, or lack of understanding that, you can't make someone with dementia do something that you want them to do unless they want to do it.

2. Identity of a carer

Research priorities for me … I'm biased, because obviously I've dealt with young onset dementia, and I really don't think there's enough in terms of younger onset, the difficulties, especially with people who are even younger than my mum: there's one guy I met who's 35 and had a five-year-old child, so the issues with a young family, employment, finances, all these things when you're not at that retirement age is just horrendous, and having to give up work early when you haven't organised for your retirement or to not be able to work is just awful. And the money it costs as well, for services, or for in-home care, for respite, for a nursing home, is phenomenal. So I can't even imagine, if you've got young children, how you'd support that.

Dementia and Alzheimer's is definitely a part of who I am now. And I don't think—it can't be with such a long journey. And the difficulties that you go through. But for me, I think it's about … it's kind of like changing it into a positive. If you let it consume you as a negative, then it's going to be horrendous, and you're going to end up ill or with depression, but I think for me it's about trying to look at the positive things and go, well, mum would want me to get on with my life. But also she would want me to use part of this to help others because that's the sort of person she was. And going through this journey, you do lose friends who don't understand what you're going through and why it consumes your entire life, and it does. But the one thing that I found interesting was people would always say, and carers, and health workers themselves as well as friends and family, would go, you know you need your own life, you need to stop doing some of this, but it is my life. I'm not going to: if you've got a sick child, you don't leave your sick child to have your own life. It is part of my life, and it's something that I wouldn't change. Because if it was the other way around, my mum would have looked after me, and it's something I want to do. I want to assist her, and I want to be able to work with Alzheimer's Australia or do whatever to progress, I guess, with finding out more about younger onset dementia.

3. Don't talk to me, talk to mum

I think to remember that they are individuals. That they're not dementias—which is a term I don't like at all. They're just an individual that happens to have dementia. That the relationship with the family's extremely important, and to treat them like an individual: talk to them, don't talk to me when mum's in the room. If you're trying to engage with mum, talk to mum. And I think it's just the little things. How would you like to be treated if you were in a nursing home. If the behaviours are difficult, why are the behaviours difficult, they don't need to be shuffled off to their room like a child, it's ok, let's look at what's going on. And some of the stories, yes, they have dementia and their perceptions are wild, and they might come out with these weird and wonderful stories, but go along with it. It's not going to hurt anyone to just agree and not argue with that person. Restraints, I just think are terrible. I know sometimes they might be … if they've got a broken leg or something, it might be necessary, but luckily where my mum is, they don't use those things. But the stories are horrendous. And just to really treat them like a human being.

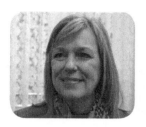

Tara

1. All behaviour has meaning

I believe that a person living with dementia only presents as 'challenging' if they are not being seen as an individual or as a person. There's always a reason for that 'challenging' behaviour. Really speaking, a challenging behaviour is a result of the person's frustration, it's about them expressing an unmet need. A person living with dementia, especially in the latter stages, will no longer be able to communicate as we are communicating right now. They are communicating through behaviour and so it's up to us to really question why and to get to the bottom of what is really going on and why they are presenting, what are they trying to tell us by that particular behaviour.

So, for example, if that person is getting aggressive, why are they getting aggressive? Is it because they feel unwell, do they have a headache, are they thirsty, are they cold, are they too hot? What are they trying to express to us that they cannot tell us verbally? There will always be a reason and for us as nurses to perhaps reach for a prn medication without exploring the reasons behind that so-called challenging behaviour is not the right way to be going.

I've heard some really awful stories about people thinking that because a person has dementia that they don't have pain and that is quite absurd. We know that a lot of elderly people suffer with pain of one sort or another; it could be chronic or it could be acute.

I was in a home once that I came across a youngish man, he was 62 years old. He was in a secure dementia area. He was in a chair; he was tied into the chair in a posey vest, which is almost like the old vests that we used to see in archives in mental health. He had a tray table in front of him, which was a further restraining device. He was actually facing a corner which, when I first saw him, it looked like he was the old dunce in the classroom that was put in the corner because they were misbehaving, and he was trying desperately to gain attention from anyone who walked past by throwing his head around and calling out. When I approached the staff they explained to me that he was always calling out and no matter what you did, he was always calling out.

I looked at this man's clinical file, discovered he was on massive doses of antipsychotic medication as well and he was really very drowsy. I looked further at his chart and I always look at the bio, so I always try and get the story behind the person when I am assessing because I like to see the person. I like to understand the person behind what is going on so I get a handle on what treatment they really should be getting. This man was 62 years old and I realised that being from the UK he probably liked the Beatles and I'm a great Beatles fan, so I sat down next to him and I touched his arm and I started to talk and I said 'You lived in England and that was the time when the Beatles were all the rage' and he lifted his very drowsy head and he looked at me and we started to converse about the Beatles.

After a few minutes I then started to question him about what it was like here, living in this particular home and he looked at me, once again very drowsy, and he said, 'This place is terrible.' As I stood up to go he reached out and he touched my arm and he said, 'You're a nice lady. Can you please tell me what I've done wrong that they are locking me up and tying me up in this home?'

Now I went home and cried. This is not an uncommon experience.

2. Philosophy for dementia care

My personal philosophy of aged care is one of a wellness model. I do not believe that we should be putting aged people into a sickness, acute care type environment. People come in to live in residential aged care because they're frail, not so much because they are sick, although many of them do have chronic illnesses, but primarily we should be assisting them to maintain wellness and enabling them as far as possible to continue to care for themselves.

Professor Rhonda Nay from La Trobe University has a wonderful approach to people living with dementia and she follows the programs—*CSI* and *House*, the Doctor House model, which is very much an investigative approach. It's that we need to always consider why and you need to, when you're working with people with dementia … it's almost like being a detective because you really have got to piece together the pieces of a puzzle to see what is really going on with that person, why are they behaving the way they are.

3. Looking differently at aged care

Yes, fortunately it's not all doom and gloom. I have seen some areas where there have been really positive experiences. I might add that some of those positive experiences comes from the really small little places out in the country areas where once again the staff really, really get to know and understand the person, which is what person-centred care is all about.

I don't know if you have heard about the Eden alternative, which was a movement started by Dr Bill Thomas and his wife Jude? It is very much a person-centred approach to care and in this particular facility there was lots of animals and plants and things around and you very often see this in the country facilities where it's quite okay for the cat to be sleeping on the bed and it's fine for the dog to be under the bed.

In this particular aged care home I was walking down the corridor and I saw an elderly lady sleeping: it was still 10.30 in the morning and she was fast asleep and she looked like she had an enormous tummy, and I sort of took a couple of steps back and I peered into the room again and the director of nursing said to me 'Oh, I wish you hadn't of seen that' and I said 'Why, what was wrong?' and she said 'Oh, she sleeps with her dog on her tummy' and the dog was under the blankets. And then I asked her if she had heard about the Eden alternative and she hadn't and I said well, you practise it.

That's how the people are and that's person-centred care.

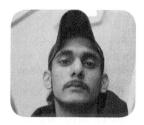

Jeremy

1. Symptoms are different for everybody

Toby: Depression, as you know, is where people get down in the dumps, and that's it. So we would call that uni polar, one direction: it goes down, and it's down. Whereas bipolar disorder, we are more talking about a type of mood which goes down, but it can also go up and get that euphoric sort of feeling. And we call that a kind of a mania. Sometimes people might get some pretty odd ideas about themselves as well, start to think that they're maybe a bit special, and start to think that perhaps they might have some special powers. Have you ever experienced anything like that?

Jeremy: Yeah I do. Sometimes I think I'm different, like I do feel like sometimes I'm special, or like I'm different, or I have powers. The other thing is I'm very religious, and there was a stage in my life where when I got expelled, and I went to St John's, I was still smoking pot and that, and for a while I stopped yeah, and I started going to church a lot and I started following God and like I was doing really well, just getting into it and my rap started to be raps about preaching and the bible and stuff like that. But then after two years, when I met this girl that gave me the pills and all that, and got me on that stage, I was sort of aware that, I don't know if you're religious or anything, but when you are really religious and you start doing bad things, you are aware that you are sinning. Now when you are aware that you are sinning, you either go and you ask for forgiveness, or you say 'you know what, I'm just going to sin, and I'm going to get rid of God's grace that He gives me, the Holy Spirit that He gives me, and I'm going to take the devil's power for now'. Even though I know that it's going to come back around, because to me the devil is never going to … he's going to give me what I want, but then he's going to take it away from me so bad, along with a chunk of my life, but I didn't care, because I was really in love at that time with that girl, and just because of the pot and pills and that. Not only that, I felt all this power just come to me like the devil was in me and I felt really possessed and I felt like there were demons around me.

And I felt like this until two weeks ago where I came out of detox and I've been clean; now I feel like I'm all for God. I've been praying a lot, but that whole stage from 18 to 20, I felt like there was demons around me, I felt like I was possessed. When I'd look in the mirror sometimes I'd see a ghost, I'd see my face really pale, especially when I was on Ice, I'd see my face morph into like a monster. The way I refer to my life is not only just with this bipolar medical treatment, but as in a spiritual side. There is demons out to get me, to lead me somewhere, to take my life, and it's really evil things out there. So I feel like I'm aware of another world that people aren't aware of: I can see things, I can read people's minds, I can see what they're about to do, I can look at a person and know exactly what type of person they are.

Toby: Is that there now?

Jeremy: Yeah, even now I can read people's minds. I can look into someone and say 'that's that type of person, that's that type of person'. I know who is around me, I can just tell, you know.

Toby: Are we talking about an intuitive sense that you kind of can read people, you kind of know who to trust and who not to trust, or are you talking about actual detail, where you could actually read someone's mind and know what they're thinking to the word?

Jeremy: Yeah, I know what they're thinking to the word, just by the way they look at me. I can not only what they're thinking, but where they're from, what kind of person they are, how they act.

Toby: Do those thoughts have any sort of pattern? Do they tend to be towards … like the other day you were talking about feeling anxious and maybe a little bit paranoid that something really bad might be going to happen, that someone might be after you, and potentially it's got some reality base, because there could be some people after you, like other members of local gangs or something, we don't know. But I mean, these thoughts that you have about being able to read other people's minds, are they normally more negative things like that, or could they be positive things about people as well?

Jeremy: Both.

Toby : What about other things that your mind might be able to do or tricks that your brain might play on you at times, like perhaps hearing things that don't seem to be real, or seeing things that don't seem to be necessarily real: do you ever experience anything like that?

Jeremy: At night time if I think about this devil-god sort of thing a lot, then yeah I can make myself, because I can see something if I want to see it.

Toby:	The devil-god did you say?
Jeremy:	Yeah. No, like if I feel possessed, if I've sinned, if I've done bad things, I'm going to feel that there is someone in my room, there's something in my room. I'm going to feel like I'm sleeping with demons; I'm going to feel like my room is darker than it usually is at night. If I'm doing good I feel like … when I feel like I'm doing good and God is on my side, my life feels hard, and it feels like I can't sleep and it feels like I'm copping it for all the bad things I've done, but at least I'm forgiven and at least I'm doing it hard. But when I've done a lot of bad things, then when I'm trying to sleep I can sleep all right, but I have to sleep knowing that I'm sleeping with like demons, with evil spirits in my room, but I can still sleep all right. I don't know, it's kind of hard to explain. That's just some things that run through my mind.
Toby:	How long have those things been running through your mind? Ever since, sort of, as long as you can remember?
Jeremy:	Sixteen.

2. When you ask me that, it gets me somewhere

Toby:	How long have you know Dr Edwards, the psychiatrist, for? Have you know him for longer than just a few weeks, or have you known …?
Jeremy:	For about two years.
Toby:	You've known him for about two years?
Jeremy:	But I've only had, like, five or six visits.
Toby:	Five or six visits with him in two years. Do you trust him; do you feel like he's someone you kind of respect what he says and you trust, or are you a bit unsure about …?
Jeremy:	To be honest, he doesn't really talk to me the way you talk to me; he just, 'okay, so you've done this and you've done that' and he writes it down. He doesn't look at me and talk to me and ask me about … he never asks me about my past or my family, or how I grew up. All these questions, they mean a lot to me, because I can remember all these things, and I can remember them very clearly like they were yesterday, and they still stick with me, even though I would have been six years old. I'm 21 now and I can still remember these things like yesterday, and when you ask me that, it makes me feel like I need to be asked that, and it gets me somewhere. But I don't know, I really trust my case manager Julia, because she's helped me a lot, not just through talking, but like if I need help with anything, TAFE courses, not money issues as in money to go and spend, but just for myself; she's always been there to help me and someone to talk to, you know. She's just sort of monitoring my drug habits and trying to get me away from it and let me do activities and find me; she knows I'm a good person and she wants me to just get to where I want to be. But I've never had someone talk to me about my past like that. Usually I find someone like on the street or someone, a friend or a girlfriend: I talk to them about it, but no one that can actually help me, give me help or medication or something like that.
Toby:	It's very interesting isn't it, the way that certain people in our lives I guess will tend to focus on different things at different points in our lives, so where Julia has been really practical help, really great, and Dr Edwards I guess at times when he saw you, perhaps he was focusing on drug use or different things that were happening at the time, and here we are now trying to really get our heads around understanding it, with a little bit more perspective. So let's just do this; let's just make a little bit of a timeline here.
	And so here we are now, and let's talk a little bit now about where you see yourself wanting to be in the future. You have been through some pretty tough times; you've had a lot of different experiences. I guess you must have had some times when you've been really down about life as well, is that right?
Jeremy:	Yes.
Toby:	Have you ever been, have you ever had thoughts of, terrible thoughts of I could hurt myself, I could kill myself sort of thing?
Jeremy:	I tried to hang myself once, I tried to cut my wrist once, I've bashed brick walls and not felt nothing, yeah but I know I've cut myself a few times but those were in my teens, like from 16 to 17, 18; I hung myself when I was 17.
Toby:	You tried to hang yourself at 17?

Jeremy: Yes.

Toby: Where abouts?

Jeremy: In my room. I just tied a rope around my neck, and then my brother came in and he picked me up and he goes 'what are you doing?' It was really bad, mate.

Toby: Have you had any of those sort of thoughts recently, to do something like that?

Jeremy: No, not any more.

Toby: Do you think you ever would do something like that now?

Jeremy: No.

Toby: How come?

Jeremy: Because I feel like I've seen; like today I was saying, sometimes I feel like I get to the point where I don't like myself, I don't like what I am doing, but then I get to the point where I hate myself, and then after that I get to the point where I hate my life, and when I hate my life I start not wanting to live my life, and then when I don't want to live my life; then I just go ahead and try to take it. But right now I feel strong enough just to say 'all right, whatever, I hate myself, I hate what I'm going through right now, but that doesn't mean I don't deserve to live'. I know not to do anything like that, because I don't feel like … I don't know, like you said I was going through a lot, I was going through a lot of doubt, a lot of weight was on my shoulders and it was just really hard. Right now I've got support, even though I'm facing jail and that, whatever. I've still got support, my mum, I've got Ursula; even though my brother is going through a lot of hard times, he's still there for me; and my dad can be there for me. As long as these people are around it's all right. But when I'm by myself it's really hard but. It's very hard.

3. Medication can be a short-term crutch

Jeremy: Now I'm starting to feel like I need some medication. Because I'm getting sick of not sleeping and feeling anxious. I was thinking yeah, all right, like you said if I just stop the drugs and maybe just clear myself out, I might get better, but it just seems like I keep getting anxious, and what you're saying about my past like when I was a kid, yeah I'm too used to that. I need to just try to, not snap out of it, but realise what's going on and try to, I don't know, think another way.

Toby: You know when you go into hospital; have you ever broken an arm or a leg or anything? No, nothing? But I'm sure you would have seen people who have; maybe you need to get a knee replacement or different things happen with our physical body. And if you break an arm, normally they put it in a cast and they put it in a sling for a while, and then it gets better and you can move it and they don't need to sling it any more. Or, with someone who hurts their leg, they need a crutch for a while to help them walk, you know what I mean? But they don't need the crutch normally, they don't need the crutch forever, it's just for a period of time. And that would be my hope with medication with you, would be that if we do use medication, hopefully it won't be something that you need for the rest of your life; that's only the case for a small group of people honestly, that's a very small number of people with mental health problems. Most people with mental health problems, you use medication for a period of time, and then you start to learn other ways of living that are helpful, and you don't need the medication any more. When I say that, the period of time that we're talking about for your situation, I would say we should pin our ears back and say, I'm going to use a medication probably for about six months at least.

Jeremy: The only thing I fear about that is that it might change me; not change me in a good way, but might change me from … like I like who I am today, I don't like the downs and the ups, but I like the way I can express my feelings when I write, and I just don't want it to change me. Like you said, sometimes I feel special and that you know, I don't want it to change me in a way where I start to feel like I'm everybody else.

Toby: All right, okay. Well, what we want to try and strike is a nice balance, where you still feel good about yourself, and you still feel like you've got energy, and you still feel like you're able to do what you want to be able to do. Now, as you know, you've seen different friends of yours, and even relatives like your brother, on different types of medication, and you've experimented with different drugs, you know what drugs are like. This is another drug, it's a legal drug. And all drugs, well just about all drugs, have pros and cons. So I think the way that we measure that is, you in yourself, you take it, you try something, and if it seems to help with your sleep and your mood and stuff, you keep taking it. But if you notice side effects, if you notice that it's making you feel flat, you don't feel good about yourself any more—some drugs can make you feel like you want to eat too much food, there's all sorts of different potential side effects that can happen with medication—then we talk about that, and we change it. We either stop the medication, or we try a different one, or we do whatever.

The other thing that would be good would be to have Ursula or other people in your life, sort of give you feedback and say it seems to help or not. That's always a good way to measure, to ask them what they think. Is that cool?

Jeremy: Yeah.

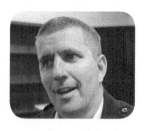

Toby

1. A clinic without walls

My name's Toby Rayburn. I am a nurse practitioner in psychiatry. I … about five years ago I moved into autonomous practice where I founded Roam Communities, which is a health promotion charity in mental health nursing, and I work with a colleague of mine, Matthew James, and basically what we do is we provide a mental health clinic without walls, a roaming mental health clinic if you will to vulnerable populations in South West Sydney.

So at the moment I run three clinics: one at an Aboriginal medical centre, one at the Street University here, Ted Noffs Street University in Liverpool, and one at Headspace in Campbelltown, which is a clinical centre for youth, and Matthew provides clinics at a GP surgery in [Tamall], one in Camden and also at Headspace in Campbelltown.

The type of clients that we focus on are clients from vulnerable groups. So those sorts of groups of people include young people, homeless people, indigenous people, people from non-English-speaking backgrounds, people involved in crime, victims and perpetrators of crime; and we work on mostly on a GP referral basis, although now with a nurse practitioner licence we can also see people who are essentially walk-in, referred by youth workers and so forth, so it's kind of fun.

Got interested in working with vulnerable groups … gosh, when haven't I been interested? I've always been interested really. It's a type of mental health nursing that requires a certain amount of creativity. It sort of stretches you to be innovative, to be entrepreneurial, to think about not just about the person that you're caring for, offering service to, but to think about the wider systems and the way that social problems interact with mental health. So it's good; it's challenging, interesting work.

2. Getting the whole picture

Yeah, yeah, so if I was going to talk about young people experiencing or people generally experiencing prodromal sort of psychosis and thought disorder, various levels of paranoia, hallucinations, delusions and these sorts of symptoms. A lot of the time when we meet them, people from vulnerable groups who are exhibiting these types of symptoms often have had varying experiences with institutional health care.

Often there has been points in their story or in their life when they have tried to get some help. They've gone to the local GP, they may have even gone to the local emergency ward at the local hospital. They may have had a crisis occur, a car accident, a drug-induced type episode where they've … where they've got to a tertiary-level type service.

However, often they've … they've struggled to get help that really comprehends or has the time to comprehend their story and their perspective and the life that provides a background to the reason why they've presented to the GP or the hospital; and so when we work with these sorts of, with … with people experiencing these sorts of symptoms, I think a very important thing that we try to do is we try to provide time.

So we try to provide time for them to get some perspective. Often they come from a place in their life where they are in a fog: they've got all sorts of things, social things, going on, or a lack of housing, a lack of access to finances.

Generally they often don't have functional or responsible people in their lives who can listen to them, and can help them to get any kind of perspective. So once we work with them by providing them with some time and some perspective, then we're in a better place to start to try and get our heads around what the symptoms actually mean. It's … it's … it's quite amazing to me how often I've seen people who've been to, you know, more than one psychiatrist, who've been on more than two or three different medications. Who, after a period of six months of working with the person or a year of working with the person, you'll start to help them to recover; and, really, medication and diagnosis, medical diagnosis, won't be a huge part of their recovery.

I've even had, recently I had a young girl who … who I worked with for a couple of years and she … originally I met her in a homelessness refuge, she then moved on through a series of relationships, ended up living with her mother, and I mean this is a girl who had a history of addiction to heroin, in and out of hospital for various crises, self-harm, suicidal, suicide attempts on several occasions over a period of many years, and she had several doctors look at her and say you've got bipolar disorder, you've got personality disorder, you've got depression, you've got schizophrenia and these sort of labels that we put on people and we try to … we're trying to help them in a kind of a way.

But the delivery of her care had been so fragmented for various reasons that no one really got their head around the whole picture; and it's not to say that I … I had the whole picture, because I'm not sure that anyone can actually ever get that. But it seemed like over a period of a couple of years the things that really helped her to get better was helping her to get some perspective, get her head around her own story, identify her strengths which she's a very intelligent young person and has been able to go on and enrol in some study and, so forth, and, to cut a long story short, now she's completely off all the mood-stabilising medication, off all medication altogether, hasn't used drugs for sort of you know a year and a half and the other day was in my office saying, do you reckon I ever had a mental illness, do you reckon I ever had you, and so it's … the messages that people get sent from the system and the way care's delivered is interesting and challenging I think.

Lorraine

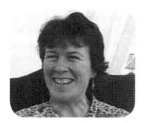

Lorraine: My name's Lorraine Nicholson and I'm here today at the Scottish Recovery Network Conference to promote my new book about recovery. I'd no idea that this book was going to emerge. It was just a very a cathartic process for me to write down what I was feeling. I had no idea that it was finally going to become a book of poetry which would journal my experiences of depression and emerging into recovery, but at an exhibition, two people came up to me and said, 'Have you ever thought about publishing? Because we think you have the potential to help other people.' And I hope that even just one word or one poem or one image may just turn the corner for someone in their life and in their journey to recovery.

Michelle: This is one of my favourite poems from Lorraine Nicholson's book, *The Journey Home*, 'Offering up the gift of hope':

Hope is on the horizon now.
There is a future, a moving on in life, leaving all negativity behind.
A surge of creativity, positivity.
Indeed a full recovery, a very real possibility.
Keep the faith.
Don't let it out of your grasp.
Hope is too precious a gift to take lightly.
It is the light at the end of the tunnel.
Grow towards it.
Let it guide you on your way.
It's a new life now.
Don't look back.
Don't let the memory of darkness eclipse your newfound sunlight.
Instead, bask in it.
Everyone deserves a place in the sun.

I don't always have hope when I'm in a dark place and things like this really inspire me and that; they're really helping in my recovery and it's really uplifting, knowing where Lorraine's coming from and also that she's willing to share it with us. Like sometimes you feel really alone and then when you're hearing people that have been in the same place or worse; when you hear how bad they've been and where they are now, it's really helpful. It really does help.

Lorraine: I've chosen this poem because it was a milestone in overcoming internalised stigma and it's called 'Unashamed.'

Say it as it is.
No need to hide the truth, to deny the painful journey made, nor to dwell on the experience, but move on in your life.
Share with others.
Being open is the only way, honesty being the best policy.
Be frank.
Be sincere to yourself.
Use your hardship to navigate others through theirs.
Grow strong from vulnerability.
Stand tall and feel proud.

It means that I've been able to rationalise the stigma that surrounds mental illness and say, why should I or anyone else who suffers from mental illness feel ashamed of it, because it is just another illness. So it's kind of coming to terms. That's why it's such a milestone and it moved me on in my kind of acceptance of self.

The printer said, 'There's a lot of colour in this book, considering it's about recovery from severe depression', and I said, 'Well, when you do begin to emerge from depression and the darkness that you've been associated with for so long, that joy of actually being able to feel colour and appreciate light is just so fantastic, you just want to express it.' It was the joy of recovering and being able to appreciate the world around me that came first and it was only maybe a couple of years later that I was able to revisit what it felt like to have the illness.

Simon: One of the things it does, is it reminds people that recovery is possible. I mean, Lorraine's a living example of that. But also, what's really important is that we learn from Lorraine and other people in recovery about the things that have helped them to recover.

Angie: 'Seeing the light in me.'

When my life's flame dwindled, flickered and went out.
You lit another candle and cradled its flame, protecting its being from the raging storm going on around it, waiting for the lull, the recovery of calm.
When it finally came, you handed me back my candle.
Together we kept watching over it, aware of its fragility.
Daily we saw its beauty and its strength re-emerge.
Now you can see it lit in the window of my eyes.

I identified with lots of the poems in it, but just being able to read it and thinking that's how I felt, especially at times when I've been ill; it's easy to look at artwork and to relate to things through poetry and artwork and you just get a better of sense of things filtering in. But it particularly resonates with me when I see colourful pictures and things that I can identify with, and there's no more powerful story than listening to someone who's been through an experience and then they put it down in a way that makes sense to others.

Gregor: The work of Lorraine and others, many others, is extremely important, not just for getting a message out but for encouraging others to feel okay about talking about their experiences. So, it's one of those things that … it's like ripples in a pool. It sends waves of encouragement to many, many more people.

Simon: We see big shifts. For example, things like the employment of peer support workers, where people who have had experience of mental health problems and are in recovery are actually trained and employed to support others in their recovery because we know that those who've had similar experiences can be real motivators for recovery. They can really increase that belief that recovery can happen. They can share strategies and techniques for recovery, so I think that's one good example of how systems adapt or are adjusting, based on people sharing their own lived experience; being real citizen leaders.

Lorraine: Individually, we can contribute to a greater understanding of the recovery process and make a collective difference. We've been to various hospitals to talk to doctors and I've spoken to a hundred psychiatrists and survived and talked about my lived experience of recovery, because it's way beyond just clinical recovery. It's not just about lessening symptoms or eradicating symptoms. It's about recovering everything that you've lost in your process of illness and reinstating your identity and your meaning and purpose in life and your sense of self-worth. So all these things can be helped by professionals who understand that process; that full process.

Michelle: All they see is sometimes a label and a diagnosis and they treat your symptoms, so if things like this— books and writing and things—let them see hopefully that it is a person. There is a person there. They have to treat the whole person and we're not just a diagnosis and a label.

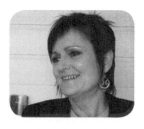

Christine

1. About the program

I'm Christine Palmer and I'm a mental health nurse, working in private practice. And a significant amount of my work is working with people under the Mental Health Nurse Incentive Program, and that's a Commonwealth government funded initiative to bring mental health nurses into primary care. So we're working alongside general practitioners, private psychiatrists, predominantly, and working collaboratively with them.

In order to work under the Mental Health Nurse Incentive Program, you need to be credentialed by the Australian College of Mental Health Nurses, and I think it's important that you're fairly confident in your practice and hold a range of skills I suppose, and the capacity to work fairly independently and also collaboratively with other health professionals. So I take referrals from GPs and basically then I call the client and arrange to visit them. I mostly home visit, so I'm seeing most people in their homes, which gives me a completely different insight into their worlds. And I focus on what they hope to achieve, so I always say to people that I'm here for them, and that my goal is to help them to achieve their goals, basically. So they work towards what they think is important.

2. The therapeutic relationship

When I first see a client, I think it's really important that they know a little bit about me and my role, and that they understand that I'm there for them. And so I think that actually helps them feel a bit more relaxed with me and that I'm not some scary mental health professional who's going to wield a whole lot of power over them and maybe put them into hospital—which of course one of the main goals of the Mental Health Nurse Incentive Program is actually to keep people out of hospital, to help support them in the community and in their homes so they don't have to be admitted to hospital. And so I always make that very clear that that's my brief, that's my goal for them, and hopefully that's what they are seeking to achieve as well. So I think treating people as equals, I come in from … as an equal, and I think that that helps people to warm up to me. And I don't think I'm a particularly scary sort of a person, most of the time.

Recovery-oriented practice

Philosophically I come from a recovery orientation. So I work with people to support them to engage in their own recovery journey. Clearly that's not something I can make people do. And so I'm—I see the possibilities for people, and try to help them to see the possibilities in their future. So on my first meeting, I'm really keen to find out what people hope to achieve in, say, over the next five years: how they would see themselves in five years, what they would like to be doing, how they would like their lives to be different. And I try to come back to those goals throughout the course of working with people so that it keeps me on track and hopefully it keeps their goals in front of them so that they can continue to work towards them.

Boundaries with clients

As an advanced practitioner, it's really important to be conscious of boundaries in relationships with clients. And as my practice has evolved, I'm much more conscious of the flexibility around boundaries when … as an advanced practitioner. So what I'm saying there is that relationships with clients, and boundaries around those relationships, can be much more flexible and fluid when you have the skills to interpret the context and the relationship. So I think—so I don't advocate for fixed, impermeable boundaries in relationships with clients when you're an advanced practitioner. I think novice practitioners certainly need to hold quite close boundaries around them until they do develop some expertise. So some of the people that I work with, I have very, quite close, I would say quite close relationships with, and I think there's quite a literature now around the therapeutic friendship or therapeutic friendliness and I think that that's—certainly that's the way that I work with people, that the relationship can be quite close. At the same time, people don't know where I live, I don't see them, I don't see people socially outside of the therapeutic work that I do, but the relationship can be quite close. And I think that that's important. That's just the way I am in relationships with clients. That's part of who I am as a mental health nurse. That I have quite close friendships with quite a number of people that I see, that I visit. At the same time, I do realise that, if I have any concerns about that, I would raise them in clinical supervision.

So, I think since I've been working in primary mental healthcare these last three and a half years, I've been much more conscious of the change in focus in my practice, and I see that there's potential for all mental health nurses, regardless of the context of your work, so whether you work in an inpatient unit or in a community service, or a rehabilitation unit, that the focus needs to be on building people's strength and their resilience, so that it's not about responding or reacting to exacerbation of illness but actually working with people towards their recovery and building their strengths so they are less likely to have another exacerbation of their condition. That they actually have the capacity to live meaningful lives, and they're able to get on and do that.

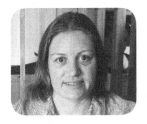

Catherine

My name's Catherine. I was diagnosed with borderline personality disorder [BPD] about six years ago and was told that I would not recover, I'd be lucky to survive it, which was very daunting. Since then I've done three lots of psychotherapy and have recovered fully. I no longer meet the criteria and I'm currently working with Spectrum, in Victoria, who work with people with personality disorders. They work with the most extreme cases and I've just been taken on as a consumer consultant, so I'll be helping with training psychologists and psychiatrists, doctors, nurses, anyone else who needs training in dealing with someone with a borderline personality disorder.

I'm also a member of a BPD awareness group who is raising awareness throughout Australia on borderline, what it is, the possibilities of recovery, what treatments are available and with them as a consumer representative for anyone who has borderline personality disorder.

It was a very long, hard road. I found a website for people with borderline. It's the first and only Australian website that there is. It's called The Shack and they support people with borderline, as well as people who are in a relationship or love or care for someone with borderline, and their key belief was you can recover. If you're willing to do the work, you can recover. And that surprised me: from everything that I had read, it's not possible and especially not possible for me, who met all nine of the criteria and was in and out of psych wards; it just didn't seem like something that could happen to me. And with their support I did dialectical behaviour therapy, which is skills training, learning to tolerate distress, learning interpersonal skills, learning mindfulness and emotion regulation, which was the key to recovery, was to learn how to regulate the emotions.

And I did stage one, which is the skills training, for 12 months; and even though I had learnt the skills and mastered the skills—I knew them well enough to teach them—I didn't apply them because I still had the belief that I was evil, that I was bad, that I didn't deserve to recover, so I didn't apply the skills.

And then I did stage two, which was a type of exposure therapy—it's called imagery reprocessing and rescripting—and that was for the posttraumatic stress disorder side of my illness, which was linked in to borderline, because I was having flashbacks and that would trigger the extreme emotions which would trigger the self-harm or the suicide attempt; and once I did the imagery rescripting and reprocessing, I no longer had the symptoms of complex posttraumatic stress disorder but still had borderline personality disorder and it was at that point that a support person said to me that 'You now have the opportunity to do this. You need to get off your fat bum and do it' and I was shocked: I was horrified that anyone would speak to me like that and decided that I would show him, I would do it out of spite. And I started applying the skills that I had learnt originally and taking steps to improve my life, get some good in my life and to stop seeing myself as an evil person and that was over two years. Two years of hard work, changing my lifestyle, changing my thoughts and beliefs, challenging everything about who I thought I was.

And then for the last two years, I've been doing stage three, which is just a narrative therapy, where I talk through self-esteem issues, impulse control, setting goals and reaching them, so that has changed my life completely, again, in realising that I am a worthwhile person and I can achieve goals, so it was the last two years that I've been doing this with a clear diagnosis. I don't meet the criteria and I don't have the symptoms of borderline, so that was a really big step and a really hard thing to accept—that I'm no longer classified as mentally ill. That was a really difficult thing to accept about who I am.

I had the chronic feeling of emptiness: it's something that is within every person with borderline and it feels as though something is missing from your soul and it is a painful, overwhelming feeling that just doesn't go away and I had been filling it with food. And I realised, this was my psychologist's last week, so over the weekend I realised that I needed to change my eating habits and once I realised that, this overwhelming feeling of emptiness just consumed me and for the first time in two years, I started thinking 'I need to cut myself. I need to do this, I have nothing else that will fix this feeling, I need to cut'. And I couldn't get it out of my head and it frightened me because it's out of character for who I am now and everything I did was consumed with the thought of self-harming.

I was watching TV and an ad came on for knives and the first thing I thought was 'They would be really good to harm myself with' and it was frightening because I don't want to harm myself, I want to have self-respect, and the pain that comes with it, it radiates through your whole body. It's like having an open wound and someone pours salt in it. It is just so excruciating and so uncomfortable that there is nothing to take the pain away. There's short-term relief, which is what the self-harming is, it's a short term 'Okay, I've done it. I can feel okay now', but there's no long-term relief and the only thing that you can do is use whatever you have used in the past that has helped for a little while.

For me it was the thought that, because I have bad in my heart, the only way to get anything out of your heart is to bleed; so if I could bleed, I'd get the bad out and I would feel better, which sounds logical but it's totally irrational.

For me, sleeping is a healthy avoidance, and I say healthy because it's the healthier out of the other options, but it's still an avoidance, which is not a good thing to do, so sleeping was the best way that I could get through without hurting myself. But I have put into place skills of realising where I am in my life, that there are a lot of things going on in my life that are really good, that are really positive.

It's actually very difficult to just sit with an urge because everything within me is saying 'Do this, just do this and have it over and done with' and to just sit with that and go 'Okay, this is excruciating, this is so painful, I don't know if I'm going to make it through this' and it's waiting for the next five minutes. 'I'll give it five minutes and see how I feel. Okay, I still feel really bad. I'll give it another five minutes' and it is moment by moment that I have to tolerate to get through it and it was last night that I realised 'Wow, I've made it through four days without going ahead with what I had planned to do, so this is really good. I'm going to make it through this' and today I'm going 'Okay, I'm still thinking about it, but I'm not going to do it'. And another skill that I've been using that I learnt from a friend with schizophrenia was when the thoughts come into my mind, I can tell them to leave and I can say to them 'Go away. You don't live here. I don't listen to you, I listen to me' and that is really powerful for separating the urge from who I am and how I feel.

Another skill is distraction. Distraction is one of the dialectical behaviour therapy skills that has always worked for me and distraction is finding something to do other than focusing on your thoughts and I went and got my nails done, I cleaned my unit, I played with my dog, I did a lot of other things, watched a movie, it was *Babe*—that's one of my favourites—so watched a movie, just to get my mind … to get out of my head basically so that I'm not caught up in the emotions and the feelings and the urges. I'm doing something else to distract my mind and take away from those thoughts.

I was bullied at school and that had a huge impact on the way I saw myself and that is one of the key things that comes out with people with borderline is how they view themselves, because they don't have a sense of self; it changes, depending on who they're with. So I was engaged a number of years ago and the man that I was engaged to was heavily into fishing and hunting, so that became my passion. It was my passion to go fishing, it was my passion to go hunting. I was into guns, I was into rifles and all these different things.

That became who I was and after I broke up with him—he was abusive and violent—and after I broke up with him I met another man who was into cooking. He was a baker, and I got all these recipes about cooking and different bakery things and different bakery items and I was into cooking as much as he was and that became who I was.

One of the key things with people with borderline, they treat people like a mirror. Whatever that person is into, that's what their passion is about and when you grow up lacking that sense of self and not having the reinforcement of who you are and what your place is in the world …

I know with myself doing … going to uni and studying psychology was a huge thing for me that, because I had grown up with my parents telling me that I'm dumb, a father telling me 'Oh, look, you're just a woman, you won't get anywhere in life', but also being bullied at school, being told that I'm a dumb blonde, and I'm an idiot and I'll never get anything right.

I think one thing that needs to be made very clear to anyone working with someone with borderline is these people are suffering, not through their own fault, not through anything that they've done, they are suffering and the behaviours that they display— whether they're manipulating, whether they're becoming violent, whether they're trying to hurt themselves—they're not doing it out of spite, they're not doing it because they're bad or because they have an evil bone in their body. They're doing it because they are in immense pain and they don't know what else to do: they are trapped in a darkness that can't be described and having compassion and understanding and looking at the person for who they are, not what they do, is one of the keys to dealing with people with borderline. And I have a saying on all of my emails that go out and that is 'Borderline personality disorder is not a choice. Recovery is' and I guess that's the key to it.

No one chooses to have a personality disorder, no one chooses to be addicted to self-harming, no one chooses to have extreme emotions, but this has happened to them; this is not something that they've decided 'Okay, I'm going to behave this way'. This is something that has happened to them and they're the ones suffering, no matter how bad they behave or how manipulative and cruel they seem to be, this has happened to them and that's where the compassion needs to come in.

Louise

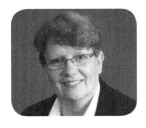

My name's Louise O'Brien. I'm a Professor of Nursing with the University of Newcastle and with the Western New South Wales Local Area Network. My experience with working with people with borderline personality dates back to when I first took up psychiatric nursing many years ago, and particularly when I worked in the community. That level of autonomy of course gave you that level … a greater level of responsibility for individual clients. And there definitely were a group of clients that were challenging for me at that time.

I like working with them because they get better. That's one thing. You can actually see a difference in a fairly short space of time—if you provide that holding, validating environment and someone who is consistent and persistent in being interested in what is happening to them. It can be very satisfying work. Very hard work, but very satisfying work.

The conversational model is based on … it's a psychotherapeutic model. It's based on individual therapy and it's based on the belief that the core of borderline personality disorder as a specific personality disorder is that the core of this is a disruption to the development of self. And the argument is that we develop self through the process of conversation, of developing language and relating to other people. And the argument is that we can only actually develop strengths for people with these disorders through the process of conversing. It's through conversation that we develop the capacity to be aware of our inner self and it provides an environment where reflection is mediated through conversation.

One of the things that all these therapies have in common is that they all emphasise a focus on the person and their inner life. They all provide a therapist who joins with the person in examining what's going on in the person's life. They spend their time exploring that together. They all focus on providing a holding environment where the person feels safe enough to explore their inner life, so that in that holding environment the therapist demonstrates acceptance and validation of feelings whilst working towards change.

All of these successful therapies have a focus on language—that the language is just as important. And that the process of naming feelings, emotions and sensations is an important part of growth; that the therapeutic relationship is absolutely central; and that the therapist actually can ask together enough themselves that they can model the regulation of their own emotions. They model mindfulness by being aware of the person in the situation by being curious about what happens in this person's life. They can focus on the present moment, and they can maintain a non-judgemental approach. These are the things that I think can be distilled from the successful therapies, and all of those things can be applied to the way that we work with people as mental health nurses.

I think that it takes a level of maturity to be aware of your own emotions and that the way that you use language. It can be extremely exhausting work working with particular groups of clients. These clients will tend to get very attached to you. They are desperately looking for someone to understand them and validate them. And when you do that, there will be a strong attachment with them. Being able to actually sit with the anxiety of that attachment can be a huge challenge for nurses. And the usual response for such challenges is either to actively attach and lose your sense of objectivity yourself or to try and detach because it's kind of scary. And neither of those things work very well in relationships with those clients. When things go wrong with relationships with those clients, it is usual that there will be some acting out. And how that is dealt with is challenging for nurses and that may take the form of things like self-harm, suicide attempts or other ways of actually letting you know that they are distressed. And I think that the … anybody working with these clients, no matter how experienced they are, needs to be in a supervised relationship with someone else. They need to seek that out and make sure that that is in place, because it's just a minefield of transference and countertransference issues. And being able to actually stand back, reflect on what is happening in the relationship is a really important part of the process.

I think that everybody has to have skills and some of it needs to be delivered in a short-term basis. And when you do work like that—say, you work in something like an access team or acute assessment team—you may be seeing clients who present with the kind of scenario where they have a background of trauma; they have a history of difficult, failed relationships; they may be extremely distressed; and they may be suicidal, they may be self-harming or they may be threatening to do those things. You can still provide a holding environment in the short term until you can organise something else for this group of clients.

And that may be that one session where you have to actually settle this down and make a decision about what needs to happen next. Or it may be that you need to see them for four or five or six times until they can actually be hooked in with another service. So it can … it's valuable, no matter how short term. Every encounter can be therapeutic.

Every time we allow these clients to feel humiliated or rejected—and they may well be feeling humiliated by their own actions because they turn up bleeding with cuts or having taken overdoses. Their sense of humiliation, embarrassment, and it's often played out in that scenario, but trying to remember that they do feel hurt and distressed and humiliated—that we should make sure that we don't actually add to that.

Most of the studies on borderline personality disorder and looking at the history of those indicate that a very high percentage of the people who do develop borderline personality disorder have got histories of abuse and trauma of one sort or another. The research on this has been pretty clear that it is about the failures of parenting—and I use parenting very broadly there—in childhood. That the child fails to develop the capacity to regulate stress, moods, thoughts, their attention, their impulses. And they also develop the capacity to be highly sensitive to what's going on in the environment because they've had to. They have to be highly aware of … children who live in chaotic, abusive households have to be highly aware of what's going on around them to be able to avoid more trauma. So they develop a way of actually relating to the environment, which they are very sensitive to what's going on. They're very sensitive to rejection and they're very sensitive to changes in the adults around them. So they're kind of keyed up all the time. And they continue that into adulthood, even when it's not particularly helpful. The research on the abuse indicates that the more complex the abuse and the more consistent the abuse, the worse the symptoms of personality disorder. So that where you have got abuse of a physical, emotional and sexual nature, you've got a correlation with the worst presentations of borderline personality disorder.

So it seems to me like the evidence is quite clear that this is where it arises from. However, there have been people diagnosed with borderline personality disorder who don't relate to a history of physical and sexual abuse, but may report a history of psychological abuse in their childhood. People that do better with borderline personality disorder are often people who had individuals in their childhood who believed in them and supported them. And that may be not a parent who's living in the household. That may be something like a grandparent. It might be teachers. It may be their friends' parents who actually provided them with some stability, some core of stability in their childhood, even though their own household might have been quite chaotic and abusive.

I think that even children who come from abusive and chaotic households are often badly treated by other people in society because they become labelled with they come from that family. Whereas the evidence is there that if other people actually provide some lifeline for these children, that they will do better in the long term. So every single encounter with a child who is in that kind of abusive cycle, every encounter that can actually validate the child and understand the child, is a valuable one, even if it's short term.

I also ask the question how come it's okay for us to be selective of other people we treat and the way we treat them when the evidence is there about different treatments? And we know how, if someone presents with something like an early psychosis, we all know what needs to be done. We've got a model in our head …

I think that we need to develop a service model for this group of clients about what's an agreed way of responding to and caring for this group of clients. And you do not see that very often—that a service will have an agreed-upon model. The research on education about borderline personality disorder is quite clear: that if you give people education about the disorder, their treatment of it improves. So I think that we need to have that in place.

I think that holding a consistent way of dealing with these clients, a consistent way of talking about them and a consistent rejection of blanket rejection of those clients and also abusive ways of talking about them, I think is also important … there needs to be a consistent way of actually not rewarding it, suggesting something else and of role models of how to talk about, think about and work with this group of clients.

If they turn up and they've presented with deliberate self-harm, say, cutting or something like that, I think that the first approach is empathic. It is about acknowledging that the person must have been very distressed to actually have done this to themselves. It's compassionately dealing with the injury without putting the focus entirely on the injury. So you can deal with the first aid that is required for the injury, whether that be stitching it up or just wrapping it up, bandaging it, whatever is the appropriate way of dealing with the injury. I think that can be done quite compassionately without a great deal of attention to it, but paying attention to how the person is responding.

If they are known to the service, there should be a service plan in place about how should we deal with this when this person turns up on a Saturday night having harmed themselves. And I think that that's one of the ways of services actually developing plans for dealing with these clients is that they should be linked to a person; there should be a plan in place, and that plan should be available to things like accident emergency departments … for people to be able to find something else to do, they need some kind of plan in place about what's the best thing to do here. And that plan should be developed with the person about what should we, as the therapist and the client, come up with in terms of a strategy for dealing with distress and acts of self-harm.

Splitting's a hugely vexed question and quite a complex process. I think that the concept of splitting is quite complex itself. And splitting is about the capacity of the person to actually split their internal world. And here I'm not talking about splitting staff. I'm talking about splitting within the self. We'll deal with that first. That often, when children learn to deal with trauma, that they actually split off their emotions from the reality of the situation. And this leads to … which is actually a very adaptive way of dealing with abuse and trauma, is to be able to disassociate from it. And that's the process of splitting: is dividing the emotions from the reality of the situation. And this in adulthood leads to perhaps a continuation of the disassociation, in which the person actually shifts their consciousness, not consciously. This is an unconscious process, where things become threatening, frightening, traumatic. They will actually split off from the reality of the situation and go inside themselves. Often this is a difficult situation for the nurses to deal with, because you might have told the patient something and they can't remember it. Or they might tell you something and tell someone else something different. We get caught up in this process because you can hear nurses talking about the patient and saying, 'She told me this but she told me that. She must be lying.' And this becomes a part of that negative process towards the client, because they're not understanding what's happening with the dynamics inside this person's head. They're not intentionally lying: they're actually treating each situation as if it were separate.

Now, often people talk about the splitting that goes on amongst staff when dealing with this patient. Now, this may be because the patient projects different things onto different people. And these people tend to see people as all good or all bad—a bit like a very young child. So that some staff get labelled by the patient as bad and others as good, and then maybe a kind of process of those staff actually getting caught up in that and actually starting to believe it—that they are the good people, they relate to the client, and they will actually do anything that they think will be helpful for the client. The other group who are getting the kind of negative projections onto them may be then resisting all attempts to engage empathically with the client. So these two groups of staff end up at odds with each other. I think that in terms of splitting with staff, all we've got to look at, how are we relating to each other outside of the patient? How are we, as staff, actually developing ways of working with clients that is in agreement, that is supportive of each other and that is compassionate towards each other? It's when we end up with stand-offs between staff, and some staff taking a polarised view at the negative end and other staff taking a polarised view at the positive end, we end up with this terrible splitting, and staff actually becoming quite venomous towards each other when we need all the strength we can get to kind of manage these clients.

If the team has good, consistent ways of working with each other that is respectful of each other's work and have got a belief in each other's work, splitting's far less likely to occur. And when it does, those kinds of teams can actually say, 'Hey, what's going on here?' But we need to be able to reflect on what's happening within ourselves as nurses and what's happening within the group as well.

A boundary is that line that is between this is what I do as a nurse, this is how I am as a nurse, these are the things that are sanctioned for me to do; and on the other side of the line is these are the things that I don't do, these are things that are not sanctioned and this is the way that nurses don't behave. Now, boundaries tend to be a bit permeable. We find that, with some clients, we can be much more friendly, close and share things with them of a personal nature. Other clients, we don't. And I think that when you talk to experienced mental health nurses, you find that they can make those judgements well about what to share, what not to share. I think that one of the challenges of working with this group of clients is that they don't have good boundaries themselves. That because their boundaries have been violated so consistently during their traumatic childhood, that they actually do not understand the process of boundaries very well. It's part of the process of being therapeutic to actually make sure that you know what boundaries are as the nurse, as the therapist, that you know what boundaries are, you know what your own boundaries are, and you know what you will not overstep. It's not the client's job to actually manage the boundary. It's the staff's job to manage the boundary.

It takes a level of self-awareness to manage those boundaries. In terms of things like revelation of personal details to clients, it needs some reflection and some planning. You need to know these are the things I'm willing to share with all clients; these are the things that I'm not willing to share with anybody, any clients I work with; and these are the things that might be on the border and that they may be shared with some clients but they won't be shared with others. The more, I guess, damaged the client is, the more careful you have to be with the boundary. It's got to do with consistency. It's got to do with being persistent around that boundary. Whilst the clients may actually want to intrude because they are desperately looking for some human contact, it is not safe for the client to have too much information. It colours who they see we are. They need us to be strong and consistent, and it should be an issue that's discussed but very seldom is.

You can usually answer questions of a personal nature in a fairly friendly manner. If someone says, 'What did you do on the weekend?', you can usually make some statements about what you did on the weekend that are broad and general. You need to have something in your head about, 'Well, these are the things I share'. Questions of, 'Are you married? Do you have a boyfriend? Do you have children?' You need to have some response that is not rejecting of the client but actually respects your own boundaries, whatever that might be. And I think as you go into a relationship with a client that might be longer term and they ask questions like that, it may be useful to say, 'Yes, I'm quite willing to share that with you or share some of that information with you, but perhaps it's more important we talk about what it is … how that is going to help us actually move on with your therapy.'

A shared approach to risk assessment

I found working in teams where there is a kind of shared risk assessment and management is the most useful and safest and most powerful. I think that many risk assessments are actually so general that it's actually difficult to individualise them to that particular client. If you know you're going to be working with somebody who has a borderline personality disorder, you know that there are risks. You need one to actually talk to the client about their risk and how that best be managed. How did they want their risks managed? What are the kinds of plans that we can put in place to actually minimise the fallout from risk? And I've worked with clients doing things like printing out lists on the fridge. So I'm getting stressed and distressed. This is the first level of intervention that I can take myself being the client. I can call this friend; I can take a bath; I can go for a walk; I can do some yoga; I can do some mindfulness meditation; I can talk to my dog—whatever the client thinks. So that there is some things ahead of time. You're not doing risk assessment on the run. We know what the risks are likely to be. And that there is a safety net for that person if they need to contact services. They should have it on a plan: who they contact in the service and what kind of response they can expect. And I think that we should also focus on when we actually do make those agreements with clients, we should focus on strengths. What resources do they have? What strengths do they have in themselves to actually manage this risky behaviour? I think that these risk assessments should not just be done with the client and individual nurse therapists. They should also be discussed with the team and they should be reinforced as a … this is a team decision about what needs to happen. It takes the emphasis from the individual nurse to the team so that it is an agreed response.

Peta: And the risk is shared then if something happens?

Louise: Yes.

Every nurse can make a difference

I like working with this group of clients because you can make a difference. You can do something very powerful. Even in short, brief contact with those clients. Even if you were a nurse working in accident emergency department who sees people coming in with having self-harmed. Those brief encounters—if they are compassionate and validating for the person and recognise that you know that they must have been distressed when this was happening and they weren't being difficult and just there to make your life difficult—I think in that kind of encounter, you can make a difference.

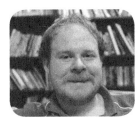

Jarrad

1. Anxiety just snowballs

Toby: I wonder if you could take us back a little way in your life to maybe the early stages of your experience of anxiety and what that was like.

Jarrad: I think probably the first time I ever noticed it it was first day of Year 7, like going to school the first day and the teacher had to physically hold me whilst Mum left and I was kicking and screaming, but before that like Year 6 I was school captain of a debating team and I was doing anything and everything. But from Year 7 onwards that first day was not ideal, but after that 7 to 10 was fairly cruisy and then I got to Year 10 and then I got to the stage where you miss this time and you have to fill out forms and have to go get a doctor's certificate and that was just more added pressure, more catalyst really for it all to start, it all build up, and then it started snowballing from there and I could miss one day and be like I don't want to go to school the next day because then I have to go talk to the teachers to get a form about the assignments. So I'd miss the next day and it just started snowballing and snowballing. I think halfway through Year 11 oh I'd missed too many days, no you can't come back, and I couldn't really bite the bullet and say alright I just need to go do this. So I had to drop out of school midyear 11 and I went back the next year and that wasn't easy, but I had to do it. The year I went back nothing had really changed. I guess I just knew that I had to do it. I had to break through barriers per se. So I got my HSC and then for two years now really not done a whole lot.

I definitely think it grew larger and larger. It wasn't addressed because I kept enabling the behaviour kind of. It wasn't cut off; it just kept progressing and became more of a pattern, so it kept growing larger and larger. So, yeah, I guess it wasn't really addressed and cut off at the knees. So I just kept progressing. So it grew bigger and bigger yeah.

Toby: The behaviour was basically this thing of I don't really want to do very much outside of things that I have to do, going to school and so forth. What can I get off socially or …?

Jarrad: What can I get out of it kind of thing. Well, it's hard to avoid social situations; it involves someone, somewhere down the line. So it's like I could got to this sports practice thing after lunch or I could not or I could just go to class. It's like what do I want to do verses what would I be comfortable doing verses what do I want to do that much that would be worthwhile going through all those barriers. So it's very much avoidance base.

2. A traumatic experience

Toby: Back in those early days when you were at high school and you started to notice this increasing sense of I want to stay away from places and certain people, I want to stay away from certain events. What was it in your body? What were the tell-tale signs that you would actually feel in yourself? What was it like?

Jarrad: Oh physically it's just the raising heart, the sweating, the shaking, breathing, yeah it's pretty much full body experience, mentally and physically. So yeah it's an interesting experience.

Toby: It's a pretty horrifying experience at times and I remember you telling me that at times in the past, I mean you've even fainted at a shopping centre and so forth. Was that back around those times, back in high school years that that happened occasionally? Could you describe what it's like?

Jarrad: It was definitely early days. It's kind of the feeling of being sick and the one experience where I fainted at the shopping centre, I was out shopping with Mum, which I tried to avoid like the plague, and she was at the checkout and I guess it's just that level of social interaction, like when you walk around the shop you don't really talk to anybody, but when you're at the checkout, how's your day and have a chat and exchanging money and what not, and I just guess that that level of social interaction was the catalyst and then I ran away with it. It was like oh they're talking, there's nothing really major about it, but because it's social interaction I started to run away with it in my head and at that stage I wasn't very good at cutting it off or dismissing it at all or anything like that, so it just started spiralling around in my head and getting bigger: and bigger the worry and the physical symptoms started to be exaggerated. I started sweating, started feeling sick and I thought I was going to actually be sick, so I started walking towards the toilets and then I got halfway down the hall and my vision started blacking out, oh I can't faint in the toilet, it'll be bad. So I just turned around blindly and started walking the other way and I just collapsed on a bench there and then.

The next thing I hear Mum running over screaming and I open my eyes and then there's all these people around me and I go oh yeah what's gone on. So it was a very terrifying experience. It took me away from shopping centres for quite some time. It was like, oh well, am I going to faint and just not shopping centres, but a lot of things as well. It was like, oh if I go here today and I start feeling sick, am I going to faint, who's going to be there and what's going on. So every little thing adds something else to the experience and then I hold on to it and it affects me later I guess.

Toby: You touched on an interesting thing there that was happening for you at the time where you were feeling this adrenal response, raised heartbeat and sweating and so forth in your body, and then it would start to have an impact on the way you were thinking and your thoughts would start to run away with you, and certainly by the time I saw you in your early 20s, I mean that was quite developed. Those thought processes were really running away with you. I wonder if you could just describe a little bit of what the thinking has been like for you with your anxiety. What things do you tend to do when you're in your thinking patterns?

Jarrad: I was very reliant on premeditating everything. I guess the old cornerstone of it all is fear of the unknown. If I take a walk through the park, the park isn't going to get up and vanish, it's going to be there, but with people I can't really plan it. I can plan it to some extent, but everyone's unique and individual, so there's a lot of unknowns involved in it. So I used to plan pretty much everything days beforehand. Like I've got to go to the doctors today, so I'll go tell Mum this and I have to get in the car and it'll be about a 10-minute drive to the mall and then I'll have to go in there and I'll look at the ground and when I get in there I'll say this, he'll say this, and I guess at the time it was my way of dealing with it, trying to cut out the unknowns, but at the same time it made things a lot worse as well because it was an all-consuming thought spiral. One thing, I need to go say this to him and then what if he says this and what if he says this, so there was no real cutting off. It was pretty much just a constant maelstrom in my thoughts, in my head, which is very unnerving, and then of course the physical symptoms go with it. When it first started I didn't really understand what was going on, so that in itself added a lot of stress to it as well.

3. Easing into treatment

Toby: So when you came to see me, we started this therapeutic journey if you like, where we've been now working together for a couple of years and if I reflect on my own work with you, I might describe it as interpersonal therapy or interpersonal neurobiology or APPS therapy at different stages. You put all these labels on it, but when you really think about what's helped, forgetting about all those labels, what do you reckon have been some of the things that have helped you to recover, because we've really, certainly in the last year, we've really made some big strides. What was it that helped in the early stages do you think for us to get off on the right foot in terms of you just agreeing to come back to appointments? I mean, what was it?

Jarrad: The whole early stages of me deciding to come back to appointments, I guess I didn't feel forced into anything. It was like we can just sit here and talk about sport or whatever we want. So I was eased into it, not oh what are you feeling and what are you thinking. I wasn't thrown in the deep end. I was just slowly eased into it. So it didn't really scare me away first day, so we started off slow and I started to get more and more comfortable and then we could address some issues. As for the last year of how it's been helpful to deal with it, I suppose I consider it just natural progression. If I say again the cornerstone of it all is fear of the unknown. The physical and mental symptoms of it were unknown to me, but obviously the level I've been experiencing it and the frequency, it loses that whole unknown thing. So as I become more familiar with it and I can explain things, this is cortisol doing this and this is why I'm thinking this, and if I can look at from that perspective, it helps a lot. Yeah, if I'm going to do something, go to the shops and buy something and I start spiralling thought-wise and I go alright I know this is happening, cause I'm anxious and I know I'm starting to feel a bit nauseous because it's cortisol pumping and it helps in that regard that it removes the unknowns, but it also helps to distract me in a sense. So, like, if what if this happens, what if this happens, it's explaining what's happening then and there, and I don't really get carried away with it. So yeah it helps me twofold.

Toby: So could we reflect on some of those steps that you've taken and how that's worked and one of the things that we did too in the first year when I knew you was we had some university nursing students actually helping you, where they would sit in the room with me while we were talking and then we would get them to go with you to the coffee shop and spend time in public places, in shopping centres and so forth, so this is a peer support. Could you talk a little bit about that and whether that was helpful or how you found that sort of experience?

Jarrad: Well, along with the whole natural progression idea of my treatments, I'm very much in favour of the whole nursing student thing because it's a middle ground. They're not mental health nurses, but they know enough to know what's going on with me, so I don't have to worry about hiding the symptoms or explaining what's going on. They just know, but at the same time they're just like normal everyday people and as you said normally peers, people my own age. So it's good learning experience really for me since I really don't do the whole social interaction thing. It gives me more experience socially and again cuts away the whole fear of the unknown thing. I can talk to people a lot easier and if I need to go somewhere, I need to go do something, then having them there I can say oh hang on, just give me a minute to collect myself here and stuff like that. Whereas normally going solo I'd probably just turn around and go home, and they can say hang on, take a minute, five minutes and then we'll go in, so they also push me a little bit. So I've got nothing but positive things to say about the nursing students. I think it's really helped me along the way.

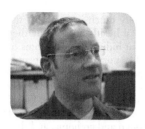

Todd

1. A day in the life

I start my day by going to the early medical unit, which is where any of the new medical admissions have come in overnight, and check to see the new admissions and if there's any either psychiatric comorbidities or mental health concerns as far as safety. The common issues that we find people presenting with would be depression, anxiety, the main psychiatric illnesses of schizophrenia, bipolar affective disorder. The people that we commonly see with anxiety are often from the respiratory areas.

2. Assessing anxiety

Sometimes, when people are anxious you can look from the outside and the person doesn't appear particularly anxious; they're sitting, they're looking around the room, they mightn't appear to be panicking. But if you look at some of the actual observations that you can do … you can take their pulse and while you're taking their pulse you can feel their skin.

When we're asked to see or when we're referred an individual to assess for anxiety we do that in a number of ways. Sometimes we use an assessment tool. When we actually sit down with the result of that and start assessing it with the person we're looking for the severity of the anxiety that they're getting, how often they get it, what circumstances do they get the anxiety in and how that anxiety actually affects them.

When people have anxiety it affects their interactions with others; it affects the care that they're able to give to other people; and it affects the care that they're able to receive from others. They find that it overwhelms their ability to do things, and becomes pervasive into their life. Often, sitting with that person and sharing the experience with them can be extremely powerful in supporting them through a panic attack or an episode of anxiety, depending on what the trigger has been.

One of the exercises that we teach them is a very long, slow deep breathing exercise and we try and get them to use all of their diaphragm and all of their intercostal muscles to slowly breathe in through their nose and out their mouth.

You can use visualisation to go with that, so you're using—depending on the person and the culture that they come from, whether they're male or female, old or young—we've changed the visualisation that we're using, so that you might get them to think of a beach or a nice calm view somewhere and so you can have them breathing in slowly and out slowly, and try and have that person be able to moderate their breathing, which merely by moderating their breathing you can often moderate that level of panic that they're experiencing.

3. What you can do

When someone's in a full-blown panic attack or an anxiety attack, it's the brain's fight-or-flight reflex working completely against that person's will and without an actual trigger that that person needs to fight or to flee from, and so when that person is significantly activated like that the best thing that the nurse can do when dealing with that person to start with is to stay calm themself.

An interesting observation, if you look at a bunch of birds in a tree and one of them flaps and squawks and flies off, the rest of them will do it too, and it's the same within people: if you get one person gets anxious and starts panicking, you'll usually find the other people around them will become anxious as well—and if you can stay calm when dealing with that person that has a very good effect on helping that person see that it … that somebody is able to stay calm and so they can eventually perhaps calm down and be like that person too.

Sonja

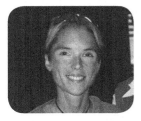

Reg: In my family we have Isabelle and me. Husband and wife. We have one son, Carl, and we had Sonja, our daughter, who died six years ago. She was a model daughter. She would come home from school, get herself something to eat, sit down, do her homework. I don't recall if I ever even had to raise my voice to her at any time from when she was a little girl till she died.

Isabelle: Anyway, she became not only a very good student but also a very good sportswoman. I think she ran her first city to surf when she was eight and she joined the North Bondi Surf Lifesaving Club and life was, as she used to say, 'Life is good'.

Reg: She didn't have a boyfriend, did she? Even right up into her twenties she had lots of friends that were boys but no boyfriends. I have to say that I'm still totally puzzled about what touched off the development of the anorexia. Was it about the age of 18 where she started going downhill and from then on basically her personality changed.

Isabelle: The first sign that there was a problem was when my neighbour came round one evening and said 'We're going for a walk'. Which he'd never said to me before. As we were walking along, he's a doctor, he said to me 'Your daughter suffers from anorexia'. He said 'I saw her coming home from the beach this afternoon and she was wearing a t-shirt and shorts and she is just skin and bone'. Scales fell from my eyes and I suddenly realised that she'd been wearing sloppy joes, her trackie dacks, yes she was a bit thin in the face but I hadn't realised to what an extent she'd lost weight. When we were having dinner and such she would only eat a very small quantity and said 'Look mum, I had such a huge lunch at university' and I asked her 'What did you eat?' and she would explain what she had eaten and I'd always found it very sensible and I thought 'Ok, she's eaten more at school or at university and therefore she doesn't really want to have a big meal at night'. I contacted an eating disorders clinic and said 'I'd like to have an appointment' and the first appointment they could give me was six weeks, hence. I said 'Look, is there any chance of getting one earlier because I'm really getting worried' and they said 'Ok, we'll try and fit you in when we get a cancellation'. Anyway, a couple of weeks later I come home from school and I just took one look at Sonja and there was thunder clouds. 'How dare you make an appointment for me. I haven't got an eating disorder. You can ring them and you can tell them that they're never ever going to see me.' And I thought 'Right, something's gone wrong here'. Anyway, three weeks later she rang up herself and made the appointment because I think she realised that something needed to be done and that then led fairly quickly to the first admission into the eating disorders unit. She got to a reasonable weight but unfortunately because she was very competitive she took on this competitiveness also into her eating disorder and she learned from other patients in the clinic the tricks they were using and started to use those tricks herself too. That made it very, very difficult. On a few occasions she was on the nasal gastro tube because it was really the only way to get actually some nourishment into her. Sonny ate quite often what I had cooked but only in minute quantities. Most of the time she said 'You're putting stuff into my food to make me fat' and I would explain to her that 'Nobody in our family wanted to get fat. It was healthy food' and she was standing there watching what I was doing, what I was cooking. I said 'I haven't added anything'. 'Oh, I may have blinked and you might have added something.' It got to that stage.

Reg: We had this feeling of complete impotence where no matter what you do it's going to be wrong.

Isabelle: Sonja's weight and thinking deteriorated, it would have been about four/five years. When she first started there were still periods where she was still fine and she'd come back and then there would be some sort of emotional upset and for some reason or other she'd sort of go back into her eating disorder and stop eating properly. And she tried to continue to do all those things that she had been doing beforehand and that actually took just far too much of her energy. She was actually in hospital and she snuck out of hospital to run the city to surf.

Reg: Yes. I'd forgotten that.

Isabelle: Yes. Those hospitalisations did help but only ever briefly because the stay was never really long enough to ensure that she would be getting to a stage where her brain started to work properly again or where other treatments could come in. Especially talking to a psychologist where she could realise that 'This is what I need to do, this is where I can get better'. Because she was usually discharged the moment she was out of danger and being out of danger was really just the physical aspect and not the mental aspect. And the mental aspect is something which, for young people, is very difficult to cope with and because she was no longer a child, so she was not treated like as a child; apparently the children they can keep in longer, and once as a young adult they can discharge themselves too. It's very difficult then to try and convince them that they really ought to be staying longer because it would be for their benefit. Sonja's normal weight was 65 kilos. In the end her weight had dropped to 25 kilos. She was literally just skin and bones.

Reg: One of the doctors said 'By all the rules you should be dead' and he said to me that he had said it deliberately to shock her, which it did, and she was very shocked. I took her home from the surgery and we went to dinner at a place just around the corner from home. I ordered a proper meal for both of us and she ate a lettuce leaf and two pieces of beetroot and I said 'Well, come on. That's what you wanted me to order'. She said 'Oh, I'll take the rest home and put it in the fridge and eat it during the week'.

Isabelle: At the age of 23 we started considering taking out a guardianship because she could discharge herself. There was very little, we as parents, could do about that.

Reg: We had lost control of her really, but she needed to have some outside authority not connected with the family who said to her 'Do this, do that' and made sure she did it.

Isabelle: Because it's very difficult when your daughter tells you 'But I will do my best, I will try' to say 'No', and, in fact you don't have the authority to say 'You must in hospital'. You can't, whereas a public guardian can and should ensure to do this and then you can get on by just being mum and supporting and saying 'Yes we can do this and we will do this together'. So we hoped that getting that would be one way of ensuring that she could stay and would be forced to stay in hospital, but basically it was too late.

Reg: I think that it did give her this idea that we'd robbed her of her freedom of action and her freedom to make her own decisions. She ran away a few times. We had the police out looking for her. There were calls on the police radios 'She's got in her car and disappeared'. Had it been done earlier when she could take a reasonably objective view of her own condition I think it could have worked, but by the time we did it that time had gone.

Isabelle: That was just the weekend before Mother's Day, well it was a Mother's Day weekend and she had meanwhile found herself a flat to rent and we had discussed it as a family, would it be a good idea or a bad idea, and we'd come to the conclusion that it could be the worst thing that she had decided to do or it could be the best thing she had decided to do. Well, what happened on that weekend, Sonny, with our help, moved into her little unit and she was as proud as punch. Really loved the little place. It was quite a neat little place. I rang after school and there was no answer. I rang a couple of times more and I got no answer so I just hopped into the car and I drove over and she'd really only been in the place for three days so we didn't have a spare key; there was nobody that had a spare key to the flat. Her car was parked outside. I knocked at the door and there was no response and there was a phone outside and I rang 000 and two constables came and they climbed over the wall and one of them said 'Call an ambulance' and they resuscitated her in the flat and they got her out on the trolley and I just was briefly allowed to touch her and say 'Sonny' and they took her to hospital and I just followed. In the hospital she was immediately put into the ICU unit. I think she had a couple more heart failures. They resuscitated her a couple more times and it looked as though things might just get better and then on the … when was it? I think it was the Wednesday/Thursday night the phone rang in the middle of the night and they said 'Would you come to the hospital?' By the time we arrived she was dead.

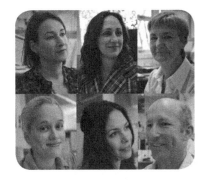

Collaborative practice

This is a multidisciplinary case conference about a client in a regional hospital. The Eating Disorders Outreach Service (EDOS) team members are discussing the client and family's needs. They are also discussing the needs of their other client—the healthcare team at the regional hospital.

Elaine: A young lady had been admitted to the mental health ward. She came in about two days ago through the emergency department. They phoned up two days ago, we sent them the initial guidelines, but I believe she came through the emergency department. She had been linked into KIMS until fairly recently and it was certainly KIMS that initiated her to go to the GP. Her family have had a fair bit of support from KIMS, and she was working quite well. Amanda will have her weight history, but I think she's actually got herself hooked and might have been 18 at one point or 19. They were thinking that everything was going well until she applied for uni, which she's been accepted now into the dietician course. So her family are a bit concerned because she will have to move down to Brisbane to do that course. I think from when she got the acceptance, things have gone a bit awry. She seems to be dropping some weight, starting restricting a bit more, has a history of binge purge, but mum thinks it's more purging now and not so much bingeing.

Carmel: Is she doing any exercise?

Elaine: She says not so much going out and exercising but she walks everywhere and she has done her driving licence recently, but will make an excuse to walk to the shops or go and do things.

Carmel: So a lot more incidental exercise?

Elaine: Mum doesn't think she's doing anything other than that, but she does disappear for a couple of hours in the morning. Often goes down to the beach, so I suspect there would be some walking there. We might need to explore a bit more about that, I think. Nothing around the laxatives that I've heard of, so Amanda you can look at the bloods later, and we might look and see what's happening there. Whether it's been purging or laxative abuse, but she certainly denies that at this stage.

Her take is that she's just become a bit worried and she's been overwhelmed, finished Year 12, which I think took her a bit longer. She's 19 now, but I think she might have repeated a year mainly because she was sick from 16, so there's a lot of pressure on her to go down now to uni. It's something she says that she wants to do but I think there is probably moving out of home and all those other things. She describes herself as, 'Going okay. I'm fine. I've just been worried, that's why I haven't been eating.'

Her mum said it's been more than that: she's heard her in the bathroom at night time and she's definitely been purging. Mum persuaded her to go to the GP just for a check-up because she wouldn't go back to KIMS. She felt she was too old to be going to the child and youth services and the doctor did a blood pressure and pulse there and her BP was below 80, so they took her over to emergency. Her blood pressure had gone up but they've been a bit worried about the bloods, so Warren, the bloods are there if you can have a look at those. They decided she was well enough for a mental health admission, which she's agreed to.

Question: Does this mean she is at a safe body weight, or the weight that the GP thinks is safe?

Elaine: No, it's not GP weight. So we're a bit worried that's probably going to be more like a 14, yeah, certainly. And mum says she's been drinking a lot of fluids too that morning, so I think a bit water-loaded too at this stage.

She says she's agreeable to stay at the moment in Nambour Hospital, doesn't like anything discussed about this discharge weight, thinks a couple of weeks just to stabilise her would be fine, so I guess we'll go through what we've discussed with her in a minute.

At the moment, parents are feeling very vulnerable. They've only got until March, they feel, to get her well, and that even though that's quite a few months off, I think they're not confident that things are going to change.

Friendships: she does have a good couple of friends but they seem to be on the Sunshine Coast, and they're going to Sunshine University this year, not Brisbane. She's got one person she knows that will be down here, but they haven't been particularly good friends. She has another friend who she met through KIMS who's got an eating disorder, so I'm not sure. I can't remember where she said she was going. I think she's staying at the Sunshine Coast. So, not a good collection of friends at the moment. Has tried to drop out of a few things. Mum thought she was joining the surf club and going down to do that, but it seems she's just going down for walks, so a bit dislocated from her community at the moment.

I'll get Amanda in a moment just to go through her diet history, and looking at her bloods and electrolytes; and Warren, you've got onto AUSLAB and looked at her bloods as well, so I'll get you to touch on that medical management, but I can probably well look at what we've done with the nursing staff if that's okay. Anything else about the family you need to know?

Question: What are her parents feeling?

Elaine: Dad's really angry about the admission, and he's not very supportive of that at this stage. Mum's anxious. Dad doesn't feel she's unwell, he thinks that 14.5, she looks fine and he thinks she's really made some good steps towards going to uni and I think he's a little bit angry about the admission at this stage.

Question: It sounds like Alice's dad is finding it difficult to accept that she's had a relapse, which this clearly is with a BMI of 14. The family would have had a lot of support from Child & Youth Mental Health Services [CYMHS], but now that that's stopped, has anyone linked them in with the Family Information Program, or the Eating Disorders Association?

Elaine: No, and I had actually thought about the skills base form from Maroochydore that we're going to run with them later this year. I think mum will go. I think dad might not at this stage, so we might need to spend some time and listen to what concerns he's got, and find out where he's struggling with it. I think he feels that she's got well and she's got sick again, and therefore someone has failed her. That's the feeling I get at the moment, and he sort of supports the daughter not staying long, so I think to engage them we're going to have to get that family a bit more unified in terms of that treatment plan. That's a bit of a concern at the moment. Mum actually has started working part-time the last six months just to give more support to her daughter, so that's put some financial pressure on them all. So they're struggling with that at the moment. Dad works long hours and travels for work, so I think mum's been at home with her daughter at home a lot on her own and she probably feels that she sees more of what's happened. We're going to have a fairly tight discharge plan with her, because she's going to go across services. So I'm just wondering whether we get a case manager from the Royal Brisbane or we get one from Nambour? I'm leaning towards Nambour because she's going to be there until March, but we'll have to have a look at whether we link her into our services at some stage.

Carmel: Obviously, if she gets discharged around 17, we would look at her for CBT clinic at the Royal if she lives in that catchment, so she'd have to be safe and suitable for CBT, and obviously has to be interested in doing it, but a good intensive outpatient treatment like that while she's trying to do her study might be great. She would come twice a week and we would be able to support her weight maintenance, post-hospital. That would be an aim. Obviously, I would have to check whether she is interested in that or not once she gets through this hospitalisation. And if she's at UQ, the health services there are very good, so getting her a new GP that she can visit on campus every week, do the bloods, support her outpatient treatment if she's come into the Royal, and keep her safe really, while she's studying, because that is a high-risk time for relapse again. Just the thought of uni has led to this relapse, hasn't it? We see so many students who are starting first semester relapsing and the GP clinic really needs to keep a close eye on them.

Elaine: The staff are pretty good—they've had quite a few patients recently but obviously just following protocols. So, there'll be no leave from the ward due to the sort of medical risk in the first seven days to two weeks, just because she was quite unwell at the doctor's surgery. Mum says that she has been fainting and been fairly dizzy at home, so medically, she needs to be a lot more stable before we do any sort of leave from the ward. So also she will need QID, blood pressure for at least the next two weeks. We've given them all the levels of which they'll need to touch the RMOs, so if her pulse is below 60, if her temp is below 35.5 and if her systolic is below 90 or if there is a significant postural drop of more than 10, then we need to get the RMO up and review her, and I've put that in the chart and they've got the initial guidelines up there. BSL is a manual. I'll get you to chat about the BSLs in a minute because I know you were concerned about some of those levels. We have really gone through with the nursing staff why it's important, and I think Amanda has probably got something to say in terms of what she spoke to the nursing staff about, and the abnormal response that you do get in this, so I'll let you fill us in on that in a minute, Amanda.

She's on daily ECGs and they've been fine at the moment. She's not on bed rest obviously because she's in the mental health ward, but we have sat and spoken to her about her right to not over-exercise. She doesn't seem compelled to exercise but she's certainly doing her usual pattern, like being the first one to go and clean the kitchen after the meals, and potter around. If there's something missing, 'I'll go and get it,' so we've basically spoken to her about her right to have some time to herself and to relax after her meals. We've also talked to the nursing staff about the need to sit down after a meal, so she is doing a lot of standing after her meals and just a little bit more fidgeting, so I guess she's a bit anxious that we've started small intake and that's probably making her feel uncomfortable. Talk to the nursing staff about how to support that using a more narrative approach, so reminding Alice that she has a right to ask things now and put her feet up and just letting the nutrition do its job. We always talk about nutrition being a medicine to the nursing staff, so I've gone through that with them and I've gone through that with Alice too, about her right to have good nutrition. Her body needs to start some repair work now. The nursing staff are going to check her every 15 minutes; and obviously post-meals they're going to sit with her or if they can't sit with her for an hour after her meals, they're going to encourage her to sit in the general area and watch TV. They've got a couple of groups after lunch, so she's going to go along to the craft groups after lunch.

Carmel:	I was just thinking, is this her first admission to an adult mental health unit?
Elaine:	It is, yeah. It's a bit scary.
Carmel:	It would be scary for her, wouldn't it? So they're aware of that, and they're …
Elaine:	Yeah. And I think also we've spent a bit of time chatting to mum and dad, so …
Elaine:	… there are areas they can go and have time out. Staffing-wise there, they're pretty well aware of some of the risks that people go through when they're admitted with eating disorders and some of the concerns they have. One of the biggest problems, I guess, is how they manage any aggression on the ward.

Also we've spoken to the nursing staff, before the meal, for her to go to the toilet, make sure she's got any books she needs from the rooms, make sure she's got some diversional activities so that she's not sitting there with all that anxiety, post-meal, and feeling bad about eating. So one of the nursing staff said that they'll set up some Scrabble games and some activities in there, and they've got a big jigsaw that they're all doing at the moment, so they're going to do some distraction, but I think it's going to be really tough on her initially. Even the 4000 meal plans are a lot more than she's use to. She's already feeling a little bit constipated; she's only been there a couple of days and she feels she's constipated. So chatting to the staff about only treat constipation if it's clinically indicated, so making sure they do an examination, they palpate the stomach, they look for signs of constipation. And if it becomes apparent that it is, then they can use some bowel softeners rather than laxatives, but we've given them protocols around that.

The situation gets more complicated …

Elaine: She's now refusing to drink. It's a bit interesting, so the dietician, Amanda, you've come up with a plan for that fluid drinking. So she's gone from basically over-drinking to under-drinking, and I think she feels anything she puts in her mouth right now will turn to fat, so she's not wanting to drink at all.

Meal plans: she's had a fair bit of time spent with a dietician, has the usual requests, doesn't want full-cream milk, doesn't want butter on her bread, wants water on her cereal, so I think the dietician, Amanda, I don't know what you went through with Lauren, the dietician up there, but I'll get you to go through that in a minute. We've asked them to do the weight and height tomorrow morning, so we actually don't have a good height for her either, so the last height they took was about 16 and now 17, so she's been refusing to have that done and they didn't think it was a major issue because she was going forward, so no one's actually done a height for a while, so we will get them to do that tomorrow morning and we will go through the nursing staff. First thing in the morning they're more relaxed, they're less crunched up, so we've gone through the nurses about putting your back against the wall, heels down, no shoes first thing in the morning, and get an accurate weight tomorrow morning so we can start from there …

Food and nutrition issues: the role of the dietitian

Amanda: Last time I caught up with the dietician she had a few concerns. There had been some low blood sugars overnight, and so we were particularly going to have another look at the meal plan and make sure that she had a good supper, and that they were testing blood sugars overnight, and providing her requirements over six meals and low glycaemic index meals, because of course that strange insulin response that these patients can have where they react to meal by having a hypoglycaemic episode.

Bio-psycho homeostasis: the role of the medical practitioner/psychiatrist

Warren: Well, if the registrar is running it day to day, I might call the registrar today, and just go through the things that he needs to monitor; and so according to our access pathways, he'll need to check the blood pressure, heart rate four times a day, the BSLs four times a day. Check the bloods and including phosphate and magnesium and potassium for refeeding syndrome, and start her on thiamine 100 mg intramuscularly every day for three days … I'll explain to him that the sort of triggers for thinking of transfer to a medical ward could be if the systolic blood pressure starts to fall below 90 consistently, if the heart rate goes down to 40 or lower than that, or even if she gets a tachycardia, because she could be dehydrated—she's been refusing fluids—so if the heart rate goes above 100, I'll suggest to him to consider transfer to a medical ward, and if her phosphates or magnesium and potassium start to really drop down.

I'll also explain the importance of just establishing the team: getting a dietician involved to come to every ward round; if possible to get a primary nurse, a nurse who is interested in the area, who is a senior nurse hopefully; and to make decisions as a team twice a week or once a week, so that the patient experiences consistency.

I find it's just really helpful to really spell out the refeeding syndrome thing because a lot of medical staff are a bit rusty on that, and explain that it's really in that first week of when feeding actually commences, and that after day three or day four you can get the phosphate dropping because the body really uses a lot of phosphate and potassium to metabolise the food, and they can actually get cardiac arrhythmia so it is really serious and really needs to be monitored, and if the phosphate or potassium or magnesium are below normal range, to replace it immediately.

She has been purging, so they need to look for signs of purging as well as, I think, having hopefully a nurse sit with the patient during the meal and after the meal, to monitor the potassium and the bicarbonate, and I'll explain that if the bicarbonates are high, she's got an alkalosis, she's probably surreptitiously vomiting. If the bicarbonate is low, there could be laxative abuse because there has been some question, I think, of laxative abuse … they need to look at the clinical signs and symptoms too, so to monitor her for the signs of heart failure. Check her ankles and sacrum for oedema, her chest for bivasale palpitations, and the JVP and all those sort of things they would normally check.

I'll send them our guidelines on the use of the Mental Health Act with eating disorder patients, but I'll also speak to them about it. Because they don't see a lot of patients with eating disorders, I think they forget just to apply the basic principles of the Mental Health Act, and it's really the same wherever the Mental Health Act is, which is, does she have a mental illness? So I usually do the Socratic questioning with them where I ask them, 'Yeah, well you're concerned with their Mental Health Act, does she have a mental illness? Yes. Is she at risk? Very high risk, this particular patient, from her mental illness, and is her capacity to make decisions impaired?' And a lot of medical staff aren't aware that when people's BMIs are down to anything below 16, they do suffer from a starvation syndrome which affects the brain, which affects their thinking and their decision-making capacity, and I usually explain to them that most of our patients are very disturbed in the decision making; even though they might seem quite articulate and persuasive, they're actually not really thinking things through. They're really focused on detail, and once their weight gets up to a BMI above 16, they tend to be more flexible in their thinking, have more insight. So I put it to them that she has a reversible syndrome that's impairing her decision making and at risk, so the Mental Health Act definitely could be used here.

Importantly, trying to get the patient onside, using the narrative therapy techniques of externalising the disorder, and trying to get the parents onside so that they can see that if she does go home, because she'll possibly be putting pressure on them, she's at risk of having a sudden cardiac arrest within weeks and that her capacity to be making decisions is impaired. I might even explain to them that the way we understand anorexia working, according to narrative therapy, is it tries to make you feel guilty for doing the right thing as the doctor. And so if you can externalise that you'll see that what the patient deserves is the right to nutrition and adequate medical monitoring.

Timing of education

Warren: I always like to take it if there are opportunities because when people want to learn and they're a bit anxious and interested in the case, that's the great time to get in there and do some teaching, and I like the idea of grand rounds because you've got the medical staff, mental health staff, dieticians, nursing—and for effective treatment you do need everyone on the same page—so at those grand rounds, because you've got all the medical staff, when you think of it, they've got so many different conditions to treat, mental health, again, don't see a lot of anorexia. I try to just give some simple key messages, which are: it's a serious illness, anorexia nervosa has a high death rate, recovery can be expected with good effective collaborative treatment, and the stages of treatment are medically stabilise the patient, which can take a couple of weeks, like this example of Alice; secondly, restore weight so that the effects of starvation on their brain are reversed, which takes weeks; and then thirdly link them in with appropriate evidence-based psychotherapy, and in this case it might be CBT for example, and that often takes 12 months, so even if we're talking to emergency departments or whatever staff, try and give the message that you are an important link in the chain to get this patient well and fully recovered, and the behaviour and cognition just sitting in front of you are reversible with treatment.

This patient is going to be in hospital for many weeks, but I think it's good to start thinking about what resources are going to be available when she's discharged, and before discharge, so we've got a good recovery plan in place. So, I'm just thinking we're going to need medical monitoring even when she leaves, hopefully some psychotherapy and a case manager. So does she have a GP, do you know?

In the discharge summary, to make it clear from GP what we expect from him or her—because they're often not clear on what their role is—so make it very clear it's to check the blood pressure, heart rate, cardiovascular status, weight every week and to do the bloods, the electrolytes as well. A full blood count, and if any of those things fall below the normal parameters we have in the access pathways—or I think in her case, if we're going to discharge her at a BMI of 17, if she gets below a BMI of 15—she should be readmitted at that point. So that way the GP's got a nice clear plan, and that's just the medical monitoring. The case manager will be networking. I always think it's nice if we can get some therapy for her to help her with the thoughts so they don't relapse.

Elaine: We're going to do some motivational sessions with her, so we can start moving her towards maybe linking in to our CBD clinic if she ends up on the north side of Brisbane when she comes down for uni. She certainly was linked in to Child and Youth in the past, so she's had some skills training in terms of understanding how to externalise, so we'll be continuing to use that; and her parents, hopefully, will come to that six-week skill-based training up the coast that we've established.

Warren: Yeah, I like the idea of just starting with the motivational interviewing with her, because we don't really know how motivated she is and there's no point in referring her to see full-blown CBT formal therapy if she's not ready, so if she does come down for the CBT, the benefit of that is that she'll get access to the treatment with the best evidence base and she'll need to come twice a week, won't she, initially for the first three weeks, and then weekly, so we need to see if she can make that commitment. It will need to be for 12 months, which is a long commitment for her, but at least the wonderful thing about the CBT is that she'll get a whole lot of tools, techniques, strategies to deal with those repetitive thoughts, or 'What if I just cut back a little bit? What if I lose weight?' and it deals nicely with the maintaining factors, doesn't it?

What is it that the consultation liaison nurses focus on in an eating disorder outreach service?

Jo: I would probably sit in and observe their handover, see how stressed they are feeling, let them debrief and just reassure them that there's plans to follow, listen to how they're coping, how they're talking about the patient amongst each other and just reminding them to be professional. If they're having a difficult day they might be forgetting that the patient's separate from the eating disorder and just reminding them if they're struggling, it seems like the eating disorder is having a strong hold on the patient for that day, and that it's okay for the staff to feel frustrated and it's important to have supervision and debrief amongst each other and with their C&C probably, or myself.

Supportive psychological processes that case workers need

Rachel: I would be happy to meet with the case manager. I think, actually, she has a lot that she can offer Alice, and we know from our experience that it actually works really well, in terms of better outcomes in the community. I think it's natural to be a bit kind of worried or nervous when you haven't had a patient with eating disorders before, because of, I suppose, some of that medical risk and especially because she came in through emergency. So I would meet with her and really talk about, I suppose, the nuts and bolts and practical aspects of what the case manager can do with Alice ... It looks like Alice is struggling with some ambivalence about recovery at the moment, and she definitely can use some of those motivational interview skills to explore some of that ambivalence, and some of the resistance to treatment. It just takes a little bit of effort building rapport and alliance to start with and I'm sure this case manager will be fine with that.

I think that the fact that there's a safety plan in place means that the case manager's not managing the risk as much as primarily the GP is. So the GP is very aware of the safety plan, so whatever the readmission weight, or BMI band and two ways and that, and there needs to be a readmission, so it's not all got to be on the case manager's shoulders. It's just more of a coordination role. So case managers I've worked with in the past haven't actually felt burdened or that that's something they've really worried about in practice, but I can understand on the outset how that can be a bit of a concern.

Kay

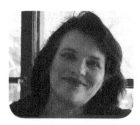

Kay: I had my first real experience with alcohol when I was 16, and by the time I was 18, I was fairly confident in my own mind that I had an alcohol problem, even though I found the word 'alcoholic' distasteful. It was then, you know, secret drinking at parties, and then it progressed to big binges of drinking. Couldn't go to a social function without consuming quite a lot of alcohol.

My father encouraged me to drink, because it's quite common with alcoholics that they like to enable others to sort of participate in the process of drinking and getting drunk. It wasn't until I married when I was 26, and although my now ex-husband was a drinker, he didn't have an alcohol problem, not that I knew of.

We had three children together and by the time my last child was born, she turned one, by that stage I was 33 and I was drinking daily. And it just basically got worse and worse and worse.

I suppose it was the not being able to accept the stigma that's attached to the word 'alcoholic', which I've since been able to overcome. I felt that sort of barrier, even though alcohol is very well accepted in the Australian culture, that sort of coming to a point where you can admit to somebody that you've got a problem, and admit wholly to yourself that it's basically the drug has beaten you; then—it's only then—that you can recover.

I went to my GP, who was involved in—quite heavily involved in—the rehabilitation of alcoholics through AA, and through programs such as Damascus. And she encouraged me to get to AA first of all, which I … it took five years to convince me, and I finally got to my first meeting.

Peta: So you spent five years with your GP making that sort of suggestion to you?

Kay: Basically living in denial, just daily drinking. Problems got progressively worse and worse and worse. The drinking also increased quite a lot.

Peta: Do you mean physical problems got worse, or what problems are you talking about?

Kay: Problems in the marriage, I think, yes. To the point where there was infidelity in the marriage; not on my part, but on my ex-husband's behalf. And, of course, that escalated things. I got more depressed and to relieve the depression, I thought the alcohol was, you know, helping, where in fact alcohol is a depressant and it only exacerbates the problem, so yeah.

Peta: Did you manage to, despite having that knowledge, to say you were still kind of denial then, until you actually spoke to your GP about it, but did you manage to work and do all of those other things in between that time?

Kay: Yes, I was … I suppose maybe the term is 'functioning alcoholic'. I was raising three children, and it is a big job. And I really … it puzzles me now, when I think back about it, how I managed to do that, and still drink daily. When my daughter was born, I had a newborn child, two and a half year old, and my eldest child was in Grade 1, so it was all the running of the house. I didn't work, fortunately I didn't have to work, but that just enabled me to spend more time at home, you know. I think the term's 'closet drinking', and that's what I became.

Peta: So it sounds to me like the secrecy was something that you identified from the beginning as being an indicator of the fact that there was a problem with alcohol?

Kay: Definitely, definitely. I think when you start seeing patterns like that, where you're sneaking alcohol, where you can't cope in a social situation without the presence of alcohol, that you … it begins to tick over in the back of your mind, you know, 'Can I stop?' And when you know that, when you can't stop, that's when you really know 'Oh, it's got me', but you still don't want to admit it, because tomorrow never comes, you know: 'I'll give up tomorrow, I'll give up tomorrow.' So that's what I was doing.

I went through a lot of mental anguish. There were times there when I thought that I was going insane, you know, really questioning my sanity. And there were a lot of other people in my life that were questioning my sanity too, because I wasn't remembering or realising the things that I was doing in blackouts, you know. When the blackouts started, that was pretty scary, because you have no knowledge of what you're doing.

Peta:	I guess I'm wondering whether there's, you know, thinking about, from a health professional's perspective, are there opportunities missed, that we might be able to pick up on? Or do you think it was all about, you know, needing to come from you at a time when you felt like you were ready?
Kay:	Yes, I honestly believe that, you know, you can have encouragement, you can have help, but until you're actually ready to … obviously until you're ready to take that step, I have a saying, 'if it's going to be, it's up to me', sort of thing, and … but I was always waiting for somebody else to solve my problems: a professional, a family member, a pill, you know. I said 'There's got to be a cure for this', and then trying to analyse it, you know, 'Oh, who's fault was it? Who can I blame?', you know. Alcoholics play a lot of the blame game. They're always looking for somebody to tag in on, you know, 'If my father wasn't an alcoholic', you know, 'It's genial', or whatever; but, oh, it's a hard question. It always comes back to, you have to hit a rock bottom somewhere along the track.

I had a stroke in 2007. I was living alone at the time. And I remember it quite clearly. Everything just went black and I remember freefalling back. And because I was living alone, I was in—they told me after—I was in the category three coma for five days before I was found on the floor, by my doctor, by sheer fluke, you know. That was just … obviously, it wasn't my time. And I did three weeks in intensive care, and then five months in hospital. I had to totally rehabilitate myself. I had … they did surgery on my brain to stop the bleed. And then I basically had to learn to walk, and I always was able to talk, you know, write, you know, all those just basic everyday things. And when I left hospital, I was fine. I could do everything. When my … |
Peta:	You obviously weren't drinking during that time?
Kay:	No, well five months without any alcohol in the hospital. But I have to admit that it shows the power of alcoholism. The day after I left hospital, I went out and bought a bottle of scotch, you know, after all that time, you know. So … and I was actually back worse. I eventually went to a wheely walker, which I've now been off for almost 12 months, and I just … I progressively got worse. It wasn't until 20 months ago that I managed to pick myself up and say 'Right. This is it. It's now. Now is the time'.
Peta:	So that's … you feel like that's when you hit rock bottom.
Kay:	Yes, that's right.
Peta:	Did you go straight away for an inpatient stay?
Kay:	Yes, I did. Yeah, for two weeks initially, and then following it up by once a day, once a week I should say, for a few months. The first time I left Damascus in 2004, which was actually the first time that I went to AA as a support group as well, I had six week's sobriety up, and they do talk about that there are main trigger times after you … when you start your sobriety, six months, three months, every three months sort of thing. Unfortunately for myself, it was just a situation where I became involved with a patient that I'd met in Damascus, and he was still drinking and, as a result, I slipped back into that mode.
Peta:	So did they talk about those risk times as being just based on, you know, every three months is a risk time? Or are there specific events within that, that they identify?
Kay:	It seems that it falls into those times, but it's more people, places, situations that arise, that you have to be very aware that that can trigger you back into a drinking cycle. And once you pick up that first drink, it's very difficult to put it down. And the difference … I think the big thing is between having a lapse and having a relapse, you know.
Peta:	And what is that difference?
Kay:	The difference? A lapse is when you might just have a couple of drinks or pick up for a few days, and then go back to sobriety. A relapse is where you basically go back to the same level of drinking. Towards the end there, I was consuming a huge amount of alcohol. It was about—I was never a beer drinker, I was a wine drinker—and I was drinking six litres of wine a day. Well that's a lot, or the equivalent of a bottle and a half of scotch or brandy, or something like that.
Peta:	So perhaps, can you give me a bit of an idea about your day, and how you might start your day, and what you might … when you wake up, did you have alcohol immediately when you woke up, or …
Kay:	When you, when I woke in the morning, I remember this quite clearly, there was a time period where you felt okay and you thought you were going to be alright. Then, normally within about a half an hour, you'd just start to feel physically nauseous and very, very agitated. And that's when I sort of I was looking for alcohol. If I had some left over from the night before, it would be the first thing that I would do. If not,

I would sort of have to wait until eight, nine o'clock, until the bottle shops. And it was virtually—that was the mission of the day.

Peta: So that agitation, was that physical agitation? You got a definite sense of being anxious, as well?

Kay: Yes, yes, yes, definitely. And very mentally, oh, you feel like you're going crazy. Smoking helped a little bit, but alcohol was the thing that would … it wouldn't actually give you a high so much, as it would just restore balance of some sort of normality. Make you feel okay.

Peta: So you'd go down to the bottle shop, and what would you buy for the day, say, in preparation?

Kay: Probably either a cask of wine or, if I had the financial resources, I'd buy a bottle of scotch. Yeah, scotch really.

Peta: And then would you go home to have a drink, or would you have a drink while you were at the bottle shop, or outside the bottle shop?

Kay: No, I would wait until I got home. It was a bit of a frantic rush to get home. One of the really interesting things about when I did finally come out and tell my friends—my family knew, they were pretty aware of it—but my friends found out, they were really quite in shock, because I'd managed to maintain my drinking when I was out in a social setting. It was only when I was in the house itself that I … that my drinking was uncontrollable. And I used to go on sprees and go a bit nuts. So they were sort of saying 'Wow! You know, Kay, I can't believe it, you know. We never saw you drunk'. Yeah, so interesting.

Peta: So you did most of that heavy drinking when you were at home, but if you were out with friends, did you drink at all, or did you not drink, or …

Kay: Oh no, I did. I had to drink, but I would definitely keep it in moderation, because I would always make sure I was drinking before the event, and that there was alcohol there when I came home, so I could cope in those couple of hours that I was out.

Peta: So you would drink about a bottle of spirits, or a bottle and a half of wine per day. And then, if you needed to, topping up with other things like vanilla essence or mouthwash or … and did you use those other things for many years, or was that just something you did towards the end?

Kay: Towards the end, probably in about the last two years of my alcoholism.

Peta: And did it take long to build up to that amount of alcohol, or is that pretty much what you were drinking from the beginning?

Kay: No, no. I would only … probably when I was about 18, a bottle of wine would be sufficient. And then when my daughter was one, so that's 17 years ago, I sort of basically started on the two-litre cask a day, which went to a four-litre cask. And that's where it sort of … it hit that four-, five-litre cask of wine a day, or a bottle and a half of spirits—one or the other.

Peta: So when your daughter was one, you picked up the pace a bit, with the amount of alcohol that you were drinking. Is that right?

Kay: That's right. I found it necessary to be in a state of oblivion. Strangely enough, because it motivated me to get things done, you know, the housework or the shopping or whatever. But I was taking a terrible risk, because you know—another thing I'm ashamed to admit—that I … even though I was never caught for drunk driving, it wasn't a case of if, just when I suppose, that I knew that I was under the influence of alcohol when I was driving a car.

I did hit a place, probably about five years ago, where my depression … the interesting thing is that when you're trying to mask the problems with substances, you don't think you're depressed. You don't think you're angry, and of course you are. And you end up really despising yourself, and I hated, absolutely hated, myself. I wasn't a good enough person. I wasn't a good enough mother. I wasn't a good enough friend. And when it takes you down to that level, where you say 'There has to be something better than this. Death has to be better than this', and you do make an attempt on your life, which I …

Peta: Have done?

Kay: I did, yes.

Peta: So there've been times when you felt so bad about yourself that you've thought about dying or tried to kill yourself?

Kay: I tried to kill myself with … I managed to get a hold of some oxyContin, which is quite a strong opiate I believe, and drank half a bottle of scotch and took about eight oxyContin. Ended up in hospital. And I really, really … I thought this is it, I wanted to die.

Two ladies that I've known through Damascus over the last 12 months have both committed suicide, both alcoholic. And that really sort of rocked me, and now I look back and I think 'Thank God I wasn't as successful in my attempt', because it's the people you leave behind. How would my children be? And also, life's so great now. All the good times I would miss out on.

Peta: I guess it would have been hard for you to think about those times, though, when you were feeling so low.

Kay: Exactly. You're not thinking about that. You just … you're desperate enough to try and find a way out, any which way that you can. And that was an option, and I went through with it, but obviously I wasn't successful.

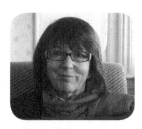

Colleen

1. Assessing alcohol intoxication

When patients come in for treatment to our service, for people who are coming in for the very first time they're usually very anxious. It's a big step to actually have yourself admitted to a unit where an addiction is treated; it's a big step to say you have that problem. So people come in very, very anxious for the first time.

What happens then is there is a period of assessment that can take a couple of days. But the very first part of what we do is very much assessing what substances a patient has been using and how recently they've used. And in particular with alcohol—and I guess this was a shock to me to find this out and I suppose because alcohol is used so widely in our society—but alcohol withdrawal can be life-threatening. And so it is really important to know how much someone has been drinking and when their last drink was taken, because we can expect seizures to occur really six hours after the last drink, that's when the onset of seizures can start to occur. And that can be before even the person has a negative blood alcohol level.

In terms of the questions that are useful to ask patients, it is really important to explore their drug and alcohol usage history in a very thorough way. But I think it's also important to say that you're doing a full assessment on the person and that you would like to ask these questions. That it is confidential information, that it goes into their file and that's where it remains, but it's important for the whole health team that's looking after them to be aware of it. And to really explore what substances they've been using recently. Ask people how much they've been using.

Now if you think someone has been using quite a bit of alcohol, for instance, it's often better to ask the person. For instance, I might say to you so would you commonly drink maybe three or four bottles of wine a day. And that gives the person an opportunity to say oh no I don't drink that much, I only drink two and a half bottles a day. So it's useful to actually ask the person if they're drinking actually a lot more than you think they might be because that gives them an opportunity to be quite truthful about what they are drinking.

2. Adjusting the pace of treatment

When patients are first admitted we really need to take things at their paces to the extent we can. We definitely have to do a risk assessment on them, we definitely have to do a substance-use history on patients so that we can make sure that they are physically safe in our environment. But after that it's important to take things at their pace; it's important to show them around, to orient them to the unit and what to expect. And it's often important to do that several times because people will come in under the influence of substances and it may not be until those substances have worn off that they're actually able to take in more about the environment.

Also in the absence of whatever substance that they've been using they're going to have anxiety anyway as a part of that. And they've been thrown into a community that they don't know; they will be with another 30 inpatients, people they don't know. They will be living, eating, watching TV in groups with patients that they've never met before throughout that period and they're very anxious about that. There are several ways we try to address it; pre-admission we try to address it. The manager of the unit where I work, which is the Damascus unit, she will spend quite a long time on the telephone with people prior to them coming into hospital. It wouldn't be uncommon for her at times to spend three-quarters of an hour speaking to people about what to expect and helping prepare them for admission; a very big part of her role. And it's not uncommon for that person to need to phone back several times as well.

3. Types of treatment

The first step in treatment is detox: you don't get anywhere unless you have detox out of the way and that's been managed and patients can come to the program with a clear head. But there's a lot more to recovery than just detox. There's a lot more to managing anxiety, managing depression, managing thinking through cognitive behaviour, therapy skills, through acceptance and commitment therapy, through physical means such as relaxation …

4. Loss

It's such a big step for people to come to treatment for several reasons. Very often people have been in denial about a problem and they become aware that they need treatment from a whole range of possibilities. Some people come to us as a result of DUIs, being arrested for being intoxicated when they're driving a car. That's one way that people are alerted to the fact that they might need to come to treatment. Some people become aware that they need treatment because physically they're becoming unwell. But I guess most people that come to mind that I've known have been people who are facing a series of losses; they may be losing their job or losing their business or losing their partner or losing their family. So often they will come to treatment because their substance abuse has meant that they've actually started to lose a lot of the things that are important to them.

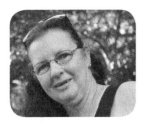

Zoe

1. Zoe's story

Zoe: The diagnosis came about basically through me moving to Brisbane when I was in Sydney. Any of my behaviours was accepted by my friends, so I didn't know that there was anything different about what I did. The first time I went to a doctor down there they thought I possibly had schizophrenia. I read up on it and I thought I didn't identify with anything that was part of the symptoms of schizophrenia, so I didn't bother going to anyone for 10 years. And up here, I didn't have my usual circle of friends that thought I had lost the plot, so to speak. So I went to see somebody at community health service. I almost didn't go, but the person I was speaking to who was on call talked me into going in. Luckily, the doctor I saw there was really good, and I saw her for quite a while before the diagnosis was made.

A lot of them were unbeknown to me at the time. People knew me by different names; they knew me with different behaviours. A good example is that I used to work in night clubs. And the DJ used to know what songs to get different personalities up onto the dance floor. They knew them by different names. They could tell when I wasn't me, the me I know. And because they didn't judge it, they just accepted it, they didn't question it. And because they didn't question it, I didn't find out until years later. It wasn't until I was diagnosed that I went and told my friends and I had the diagnosis clarified by a specialist in Sydney. So when I came back and I said, oh I've got—at that stage it was called multiple personality disorder—they just laughed and said, we knew that, we've known that for years, we thought there was something important. So yeah, the reaction I got was quite different to what I expected.

Mostly losing time is one. Not remembering having been places. Sometimes the problem isn't so much for me, it's for other people. When I first applied to get some training to become a counsellor, the social worker I spoke to said because I don't remember going to school, I should do numeracy and literacy. And I couldn't explain to her that just because I couldn't remember it, didn't mean I couldn't do it. I said I've probably got books at home with words in it that you would die at. I just don't remember going to school, I don't remember learning. But the knowledge is in there. So sometimes the issue isn't with me, it's with other people and how they handle it.

I don't remember going to school. Actually, the things I do remember about school have nothing to do with school. They're outside things. I remember running the oval because I wanted to be a long-distance runner. And the same with my life as a child: I don't remember a lot of indoor stuff. It's only a little bit, but I remember a lot of outdoor stuff.

Margaret: Zoe, a lot of people who have dissociative identity disorder have a past that had trauma in it. Was that the case for you?

Zoe: Yeah. I don't remember a lot of it. I go by what family members tell me, flashbacks I've had, even some things that the particular people or one of the particular people admitted. Yeah, it was, like they say, the repeated abuse on a daily basis. I don't remember school because my friend from high school tells me I was picked on every day and bullied every day. Apparently I was pushed down the stairs a few times. I don't remember that at all.

The best way to explain it is if you've got, say, you're having a conversation with someone and you're talking about a movie you saw, and a third person taps you on the shoulder and says, oh yeah but don't forget about the character that did that. Then they go away again. That can happen. So I can be talking to you and it could be happening now. I won't remember all of this. And the end of this, I won't remember all of this. It's almost like standing in the background and if I'm not saying something or if I've forgotten something, they might just come through and quickly say it and go away.

If Linda came out now, I would behave like a 10-year-old; my body language would be that of a 10-year-old, and apparently my eyes pin and that's not something that a person can control—the pupils pinning. For all intents and purposes, it's a 10-year-old being silly.

Margaret: Zoe, another thing that you won't mind me talking about is that you used to self-harm quite a bit. Could you talk about that?

Zoe: Again, it's another thing I don't actually remember doing. I'd be having a shower, my arm would sting, and I'd look down and there would be a burn there. I never called it self-harm before I actually got into the mental health area.

Margaret: What did you call it?

Zoe: I just called it burning myself or cutting myself. And while it was annoying having a scar on my arm, for me at the time, the benefits outweighed the harm because for a couple of days I wouldn't lose time. I'd feel good, I wouldn't feel guilty, I wouldn't feel panicky. Every night at nine o'clock I get scared; in those days it was sheer panic. So that wouldn't happen for a couple of days. The physical wounds were superficial. I'd already had scars on my arms from dog bites and fence scratches when I worked at the RSPCA, so I wasn't this sort of prissy person who didn't want a scar on my body, so I didn't particularly care. I wish I had known more about tattooing back then; I would have had at least pretty arms, if not scarred arms.

I can sort of look back and think, well, I obviously did it to get through the day because if I got up and the burn would already be there, even though I didn't remember doing it. But for a couple of days I'd feel good. I wouldn't … the official term is switching, but my term back then was dipping out because I just dipped out. So I wouldn't dip out. I wouldn't switch. I seemed to cope with things better for a couple of days. I have no idea why that is. I still don't know the technical connection. But maybe while I felt the sting of the burn on my arm I felt real. I felt like I was part of the world, that I was here. So, for me, I didn't consider it self-harm. It was just something that happened that was a small price to pay because it was only superficial.

It was a superficial mark on my body that let me get by three or four days. And I didn't feel guilty about it until the first time I went into hospital. The nurse came up to me and said, we won't tolerate any attention-seeking behaviour here. That confused me because I was performing and my whole image was to gain attention so that when I performed on stage people would look at me. So I said to her, what, I can't dance? She got confused and said, no I meant the self-harm. And I said, oh that, don't worry: if I do that you won't know about it. I said, I don't show people.

The thing that got me, that I discovered, and it's particularly with this one, she was an older nurse, is that soon as someone even made any attempt to cut themselves, she'd be all over them. So she was actually teaching them that if they want her attention straight away, do something attention-seeking like break a cup and threaten to slash your wrist. And if you didn't do anything to say I need help, she wouldn't come near you.

2. Triggers for switching

Zoe: … because I don't know a lot of it, but basically switching from one personality to another. One of the main things I found out when I got diagnosed and saw the specialist is I wasn't the first born. I'm basically just one of the personalities. So I can't even regret having the condition because I wouldn't be the me I am now. That's probably why I remember all the outdoor stuff because my job was to have fun. If it wasn't fun I wasn't there, so that's why I don't remember all the bad stuff. But basically, switching is when, whoever I am, closes my eyes and when I wake up it's two hours later or two days later. Somebody else has obviously come out and did something.

I've got lots of triggers. This wind is a trigger. It makes me want to go out and walk around in it. So if I'm at home, and this sort of weather comes up, I get itchy and want to get out and about.

Margaret: And do you switch?

Zoe: Not so much now, but there would have been a time where if I had of defied that urge, then I would have switched. I guess an example was I went somewhere to do some training and I wasn't comfortable. And I always push myself to do things. I try not to give up on things. So I pushed myself and stayed in the situation, which wasn't good for me. The only way I can explain it is that I blinked and opened my eyes and I was standing at the bus stop. Now, at that stage I had known what my diagnosis was so it didn't freak me out. And I just thought, well, somebody got me out of there.

3. Cooperation is my goal

Margaret: What's been the aim in the therapy for you?

Zoe: Mainly, I guess, just cooperation amongst, in what they call the system of personalities. When I first started talking to my doctor, one of the subjects that came up was integration, which in a lot of the books says that's what the goal is.

Margaret: What did it mean for the others if they were to be integrated?

Zoe: Well, a kind of death really, because they wouldn't be who they were. And while logically it would mean all the parts coming together to becoming one, but what people don't realise is, that's again, a new one. It might be just one personality but it's nothing like the personalities that have been before it. I think people think that you do your integration and you internally hug each other and become one and then, yay, life's rosy. But it's not because you've got to learn to deal with behaviours that you've never known, emotions you've never known. I can have all the emotions—I can feel anger, happiness and all that—but I can only feel them to a certain degree. I can be angry to a certain point. After that, the angry one takes over. If I integrated that, I haven't had a life of dealing with that sort of anger. So what sort of person would I be? I don't want to be the sort of person that walks around so angry that I pick fights with people or that I suddenly hate the world.

Margaret: So you were saying the aim for you in therapy then is to learn cooperation?

Zoe: Yeah, cooperation with the others. And that's worked: I don't lose time as much as I used to. I used to get headaches because the others would be trying to get out all the time. The only way I can liken it is to, you know, several people trying to leave the same doorway and everyone getting squished in the doorway. I think that used to happen.

I understand you need to come out or you need to do something, but can you wait 'til we get home because I need to concentrate on catching the buses. It didn't always work, but sometimes it would be instant. The headache would be instantly gone and my eyes would be clear and that sensation of everyone crowding around me would be gone. I'd get home and I'd keep my promise. I'd have a shower and I'd let my emotions go, you know, and if they'd want to come out and cry or rant, rave or whatever they wanted to do.

Margaret: So what's your final word, Zoe?

Zoe: I think my final word would be, whether you're a nursing, doctor, counsellor or any profession like that, is try not to be judgemental. It doesn't matter what the person is going through at the time, everyone is going to come from their own perspective. But someone who self-harmed or someone who is dissociative; they've got a background. And if you don't know it how can you judge why they're behaving that way? Someone who is crying might be crying because they just lost someone in an accident the day before. So who knows why they're behaving the way they do. Sit down and ask them.

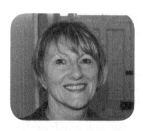

Jay

1. Mental illness and violence

My name's Jay Hendricks. I'm a registered nurse. I currently work at the Queensland Health Victim's Support Service and my role there is as both a clinician and as the assistant manager.

The Victim's Support Service is a state-wide service. It provides support, counselling, information and basically it helps people to negotiate or navigate through the forensic mental health system. We work with victims of serious violence where the person who has committed the violence has a mental illness and is diverted from the criminal justice system into the mental health system.

We have a very broad definition of victims … we have people who are the direct victims or family members of the direct victims; people who are impacted upon through witnessing or have been a part of what happened; and also we have what perhaps is a little unusual, is that we actually provide support to the offender's family as well. So we realise that the offender, who is actually a mental health patient, their family also is in need of support because they not only have a family member who has a mental illness and the stigma attached to that, but the person has committed a serious violent offence.

I think that in general the public have a perception of mentally ill people and violence that is quite disproportionate … If we took the newspaper and took a blue marker and we marked out all of the information that was negative and we marked out all of the information that was none of our business in red, we'd have very little left. If we took a green marker and we highlighted those offences that were reported by people having a mental illness, we'd have most of the time no green at all or very little. So when you actually saw the green appear it would stand out because it's such a rare event and certainly that's how it is. Once the media do get hold of a significant violent event where the person may have mental illness, not necessarily that they do but may, then it tends to be front page news and certainly it causes lot of angst amongst the general community.

For the most part, we can provide support for the victims in helping them understand mental illness, to talk to them about what mental illness is and what someone can expect with different types of mental illness. We try and help them understand about psychosis and some of the beliefs that people who have a psychotic illness can hold and how the beliefs are fairly intractable, they're quite systematised, and that the thinking process is not the same as someone without the mental illness who might be able to think rationally and logically and attribute meaning a particular way. So it's often about helping them understand the complexities of what mental illness is and how that impacts on people's behaviours.

We provide support to victims for as long as they require it, so we don't have an end date with them and we try and engage with them. Our service doesn't treat victims as if they were patients. In fact, they are just ordinary people who are reacting to an extraordinary event and usually they're dealing quite well with it.

A key message I suppose is to say that the number of people with a mental illness who commit serious violence is so small in comparison to the violence committed in the community in general and it's all well and good with hindsight to say 'We should've done, we could've done, why didn't we do?' What I think is the biggest factor that has become apparent through working in our service is communication, and certainly the necessity to hear the bigger picture stories. So when you're conducting assessments, whether they're risk assessments or general assessments, it's about really looking at what collateral information you can get and who you can get that from, and how you can use that information once you have it and what are the limits to confidentiality, but also there's never a limit on listening.

2. It's about balance

All of our staff are mental health professionals so we've all worked within the system for an extended period of time in one form or other.

We can use that skill to have an objective view on what's happened. So we don't sort of engage and take sides. We try and balance the information so that we can actually help the victim work through what they're going through and their trauma and also to provide an understanding of mental illness and the process of how that works.

Clinically we use a lot of our skills perhaps a little more, not covertly, but it's a bit like driving a car. You don't really think about what you're doing, you just do it and we use it more conversationally. So our assessment process of people is done very conversationally and we look at people's needs in regards to their immediate needs; so to be safe, to make sure that they have all the information that they require, to ensure that they have access to appropriate supports—we do a lot of referral to other psychological services if we feel the people are significantly traumatised and would benefit from that.

But in general we help people to work through some of their grief. We help them to sort of normalise and to work through the situation and we also look at providing some counselling in terms of their response to trauma.

I think communication is very important and can have a significant impact on relationships between victims and family members in the community. It's really important I think to have really good communication pathways and to engage with people. I think when you're looking at doing a risk formulation it's vital to not just have the self-report of the patient, clinical history and background, sort of general collateral, but I think it's really important to actually talk to the family and carers and other social networks I suppose or people who know the person well, to actually get a much broader picture of what's been happening for them in the community leading up to their hospitalisation and also how can you then look at ensuring that you manage the risks when you're returning them back to the community.

I think it's about finding that balance where you are working to keep the community safe but also to ensure that the patient is not put in a position where they are likely to reoffend or put themself in a situation where they might become more distressed and is a possibility they may commit a further offence.

3. Everyday people, extreme circumstances

We don't have a specific model in our service that we work from in terms of our clinical care. We adopt I suppose different models of care for each individual. It really is very dependent on what it is that that person requires at that time and we don't treat our clients as patients; they're just everyday people who are going through difficult circumstances and I think if we were to try and adopt particular models then it would actually change the focus of our service.

We try to formulate an assessment in terms of what is it that this person needs at this point in time from their perspective and what are their understandings of what has happened to them or to their family member. After that, it's really looking at what are their support networks, who do they rely on, how are they coping in themselves? Are they sleeping well, are they looking after themselves, are they having poor sleep, nightmares, hypervigilance and concerns that you start to associate with symptoms of a traumatic experience, and looking at how you can assist them. Are they depressed, which is a normal reaction, and how do you actually support people and help them through those processes. So I think we look at a hierarchy of needs and we generally work with people to address those.

Working with victims of mentally ill offenders (sic) is obviously a speciality and it's not for everybody. I think having life experience and good understanding of mental illness and how mental illness progresses and also of the mental health system and how services are provided to people with mental illnesses is vitally important. Working with people who have significant distress and anger and trauma, you need to have a very good sense of self and able to self-reflect and to be able to be professional, but also to be objective within your own humanity really.

So I think people who come to work in the area, I think it's a genuine desire to assist people when again they're in a marginalised proportion of our community, because victims do tend to be kind of left behind. We find that the focus is very much on the patient because that's where all the services are and that's where the focus is, not about the victims. So I guess it's that working from an advocacy model as well and being very clear about your role with that.

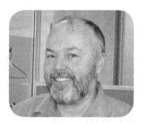

Bill

1. Culture clash—working within different philosophies

The complexity of working in forensic mental health services within a prison system as opposed to a hospital system is the contrast of our role within the service. When we work in a hospital we are the predominant providers of care: the nurses and the doctors determine the way that the day goes for the client. In the prison system, where they are responsible for our patients (who are their inmates) and so we are invited into the prison to provide services to their customers, and from that perspective our role changes because we are invited in. We provide service at their whim, so to speak, so often access to patients is very difficult. The patients are part of the prison establishment and they have to relate to all of the prison roles, activities and the security systems that we have got in the prison, so access is hard. Some of them are in their cells in prison wings and some of them are in prison hospitals, but those prison hospitals, for the lay person, they are just another bunch of cells that happen to be in one building called a hospital. We have to deal with the philosophies of care that relate to both our prison service and our health service and that is an area of conflict for me and it is an area of conflict for a lot of nurses. Our role as nurses is to build a relationship. My training in both forensic and in mental healthcare was that the relationship is the key thing; the relationship is the key to all nursing, and so we build a relationship of trust. We have continuity, we have the same providers speaking and building and building on the previous contexts and we build that trust. Whereas, in the prison service the philosophy is that you don't create a relationship with your client because a relationship is something that can be breached and a relationship becomes a chink in security, so while we are trying to build relationships, they are trying to stop us having relationships, not actively so, but the philosophy is different.

The prison service often doesn't have enough staff, or staff is doing other duties and you can't get them out, and we have periods of time where we would expect to spend an hour with a client and we only may get five minutes. We can't walk through the prison and identify patients who may be at risk. During our normal nursing observation, we will watch someone in a ward situation who is withdrawing, who is slowly deteriorating, whose behaviour is just subtly changing, and as nurses we would pick that up. Those clients don't get picked up early because the prison officers don't have that training, so often they get brought in an advanced state of psychosis to us or they get an advanced state of depression. Whereas, if they are in a ward situation we would pick that up by sitting having coffee with them, walking with them, sitting maybe in a quiet room, in a lounge with another group of people picking them up and watching the corrections; we don't get that ability in the prison.

It is also our role in the prison to educate officers, prison officers who have their own training. It is to build relationships with the prison officers to give them information to sort of identify when the patient is deteriorating or not deteriorating. That also has a conflict of confidentiality. The role of prison officers is to collect data, to collect information and they keep their own files. They have their files for different reasons and so keeping our own information confidential is difficult, but there are ways around it where you can talk and you can identify things to look for and it is about using every opportunity.

Every prison is different and I think mental healthcare in prisons is improving all of the time, but the opportunity to sit with your patient often doesn't happen without having a security person in the same room or outside the door, so we use those opportunities. We use meal times, when you are walking from A to B, we use exercise yard time to get amongst the clients, and the good nurses are the nurses that talk to the patients and not to each other. You often see excellent nurses who position themselves in amongst the exercise yard where clients can come up to them and talk in confidence. We used to watch one nurse who always used to take two chairs into the exercise yard, put them against the sale boards, sit down in one and he would just sit there and the second chair was never empty and I learnt a lot from that, where you just make yourself available—you use opportunities. Clients are desperate to talk. There is a prison culture that often having to talk to you when you sit down in an exercise yard or a common area, where being seen talking to staff is seen as a weakness, in the culture of the other prisoners and their status …

I always think there are two teams in the prison. There is a the green team and the blue team and everybody has a role in a team; and the prison officers have their role and the inmates have their role and the people in civilian clothes like the health professionals and the various health people coming in are like the referees and the officials. You have a role to play in a team and it is not the done thing to be seen talking to prison officers and it is often not the done thing to be spending time talking to nurses. We have a great role in breaking that down and moving amongst the patients or the inmates and making ourselves available. There are opportunities there for good nurses to take it and you have just got to look for every opportunity to talk to your patient or your client.

2. Treat the person, not the crime

One of the things that I often find distressing working in the acute admitting area in the prison is that you will get someone who has come into the prison who has been charged with some offence that is pretty awful, for want of a better description—an offence where a child may be killed or a family member may be killed or something like that—and what you are looking at is the person as your client who is in tremendous distress. They are bewildered; they have got only a little bit of comprehension of what they have done. They may have killed their daughter and at times I am thinking back when I have seen young mothers who have come in who have killed their own children while they have been psychotic and while they have been unwell. Everybody treats them like a leper, no one touches them; no one is allowed to talk to them. The only people that have physically touched them were the people who have clipped their handcuffs on them and often behind their backs when they are being transported from A to B and these people actually need physical contact.

Often what you see is you see this person standing in front of you trembling and they are bewildered that they have just been told they have killed their child and some of them don't even remember they have done it and all they need is a big hug and, you know, I think many nurses have been chastised. 'You can't touch the patients, you can't' and what we have learnt over a period of time is that it is okay and the way I go about it is ... in the prison there are cameras everywhere and what I tend to do is go and stand underneath the camera. You would give someone a hug and you would sort of put your arms around them where your hands are up, where they are always exposed to the camera, or you touch them on the arm, constantly holding their hand between their hand and their elbow where everybody can see openly what you are doing. You know you do this in the prison and very quickly prison officers come running and 'you are not allowed to touch the client, you know. Are you passing contraband or anything like that' and we constantly do those things to a point where people start accepting that as normal behaviour. When we set up that unit, which was a women's high-dependency unit, we started going and having morning tea with our patients and sit at the table in the common area and have a cup of tea and sit and talk with our patients and the prison officers found that quite disturbing that we would sit down and drink with the patients. But once we started doing it and after about three or four months the prison officers started joining us and often you would have a big round table where there would be two or three patients, a couple of nurses and a couple of prison officers. Then we started playing cards with them and then we started playing volleyball with them and so, by example, and by being inclusive, you can actually create the change and you can create an environment. Then, you know, we sit down and it is such a joy to sit down and look out into the prison wing at these horrible concrete walls and metal tables bolted to the floor then you would see a nurse and two patients and a prison officer playing scrabble together and you would think 'yes, we are getting it right'. I remember Christmas day and the first time in that unit we went and made up lolly bags and we put them in all of the inmates' cells while they were out exercising and got caught doing it and we got admonished and dragged before the governor; and the following year it was allowed. So progress does happen, but it is up to us to make it happen.

3. Prison is an awful place

Prison is an awful place: it is cold, it is hot, it is never just right. It is noisy, the gates are made to clang, the halls always echo, there is no privacy and I often sit in the courtyard with the patients and they have got these high walls that are about 15 and 16 feet tall. The only thing they can see are these planes going away or going somewhere without them, so by going to work you actually make a difference. You make a difference because they trust you. You are someone fresh to talk to, you have got an attitude of wanting to listen to them and it is not as though you have to listen to them, and it is incredibly rewarding just by going to work. You make a difference by going to work and I think that is what you get out of it, for me anyway.

One of the things that impressed me is that often it is one of the safest areas to work in. People are very fearful of people who have committed crimes and fearful of forensic and often it is a fear of the unknown, but our clients because of the nature of what happens, there are really good practices for safety and you have got to maintain the practices for safety. There are a lot of protections in place so it is not a place to be fearful of; it is a great place to learn.

I had preconceptions that totally went out the window. I thought prison would be full of a lot of bad people and what I found was it was full of a lot of good people who have done some bad things but they are not bad people. They are people I would have in my home. They are people that I would trust to drive my car to do this, to do that. You know, that was the thing that surprised me the most, they were people that you can trust.

I have seen lots of people who have been caught stealing food, caught breaking into buildings for somewhere to sleep. They are not bad people. We make such a difference and I think that one of our roles is because we can, particularly in my role at the moment. My role is to get a solution and as long as we professionally keep within our boundaries, as long as we maintain our risk assessment, as long as we are allowing people to go home into a safe environment with the protective situations, then we can do anything.

Chapter alignment	Story
Setting the scene/the underlying philosophy behind the work	**Story 1** **Makhala's story** Resilience
	Story 2 **Jennifer, Anne and Christine's story** Cultural and social inclusion
	Story 3 **Toby's story** Being authentic
	Story 4 **Bernie's story** The lived experience
	Story 5 **Jean's story** Carers
	Story 6 Recovery
	Story 7 Clinical supervision: Learning about self and other
Chapter 3 *Historical foundations*	**Story 1** **Claire's story** How mental health has changed
Chapter 12 *Intellectual disabilities*	**Story 1** **Lisa's story** Experiencing a major life transition
	Story 2 **Mike's story** Facilitating empowerment
Chapter 13 *Disorders of childhood and adolescence*	**Story 1** **Gordon's story** Fatherhood
	Story 2 **Rachel's story** Relating to young people
Chapter 14 *Mental disorders of old age*	**Story 1** **Nadine's story** Having a parent with a mental illness
	Story 2 **Tara's story** Humanising dementia care
Chapter 15 *Schizophrenic disorders*	**Story 1** **Jeremy's story** Beliefs and perceptions

Chapter alignment	Story
	Story 2 **Toby's story** Providing an accessible service
Chapter 16 *Mood disorders*	**Story 1** **Lorraine's story** A creative consumer advocate
	Story 2 **Christine's story** Primary mental health care
Chapter 17 *Personality disorders*	**Story 1** **Catherine's story** Reframing personality disorder
	Story 2 **Louise's story** On conversational models
Chapter 18 *Anxiety disorders*	**Story 1** **Jarrad's story** Containing fear
	Story 2 **Todd's story** Consultation liaison
Chapter 19 *Eating disorders*	**Story 1 TBC** **Sonja's story** Finding strengths
	Story 2 Collaborative practice
Chapter 20 *Substance-related disorders and dual diagnosis*	**Story 1** **Kay's story** The social and physical impacts of alcohol
	Story 2 **Colleen's story** Health education as core to mental health nursing
Chapter 21 *Somatoform and dissociative disorders*	**Story 1** **Zoe's story** Living with multiple selves
Chapter 22 *Forensic mental health nursing*	**Story 1** **Jay's story** Being non-judgemental
	Story 2 **Bill's story** Cultivating a therapeutic milieu

Printed in Singapore by Markono Print Media Pte Ltd